Study Guide for

INTRODUCTION TO HUMAN ANATOMY AND PHYSIOLOGY

Second Edition

■ ■ ■

Eldra Pearl Solomon, PhD
Mical K. Solomon, LMT
Karla Solomon, RN

SAUNDERS
An Imprint of Elsevier

SAUNDERS
An Imprint of Elsevier
11830 Westline Industrial Drive
St. Louis, MO 63146

Executive Vice President, Nursing and Health Professions: Sally Schrefer
Acquisitions Editor: Tom Wilhelm
Senior Developmental Editor: Jeff Downing
Developmental Editor: Eric Ham
Senior Designer: Kathi Gosche

Study Guide for

INTRODUCTION TO HUMAN ANATOMY AND PHYSIOLOGY

Second Edition

■ ■ ■

USING THE STUDY GUIDE

■ ■ ■

Learning anatomy and physiology has been compared to learning a new language. To understand how the body is constructed and how it functions, you must learn the language used by health professionals. The exercises included in the *Study Guide for Introduction to Human Anatomy and Physiology* are designed to help you learn both the words and the concepts presented in the textbook, *Introduction to Human Anatomy and Physiology,* by Eldra Pearl Solomon, Ph.D. Working through the exercises, diagrams, and crossword puzzles will help you test your mastery of the material and gain both knowledge and confidence.

Follow the following steps to help you use this Study Guide effectively.

1. Read the Outline presented at the beginning of the chapter. The outline reflects the organization of the corresponding textbook chapter and provides you with an overview of the material in the Study Guide chapter.

2. Read the Learning Objectives and refer back to them frequently as you work through the chapter exercises. The Learning Objectives tell you what you need to do to demonstrate mastery of the material.

3. Answer the Study Questions provided for each section. After you complete a section, check your answers in the Answer Key at the back of the book. If one or more of your answers are incorrect, reread the corresponding sections in the textbook.

4. Label the diagrams that are provided in appropriate sections throughout the Study Guide. To check the accuracy of your labels, consult the corresponding labeled diagram presented in the textbook.

5. When you feel confident that you have learned the material in the chapter you are studying, check your level of mastery by completing the Chapter Test at the end of the chapter.

6. To build your confidence even more, complete the Crossword Puzzle provided for the block of chapters you are studying. Answers are provided in the Answer Key.

CONTENTS

■ ■ ■

Chapter

1

INTRODUCING THE HUMAN BODY

■ ■ ■

Outline

Introducing the Human Body
I. The body has several levels of organization.
II. The body is composed of inorganic compounds and organic compounds.
III. The body systems work together to maintain life.
IV. Metabolism is essential to maintenance, growth, and repair of the body.
V. Homeostatic mechanisms maintain an appropriate internal environment.
VI. The body has a basic plan.
   A. Directions in the body are relative.
   B. The body has three main planes.
   C. We can identify specific body regions.
   D. The body has two main cavities.
   E. It is important to view the body as a whole.

Learning Objectives

After you have studied this chapter, you should be able to:

1. Define anatomy and physiology.
2. List in sequence the levels of biological organization in the human body, starting with the simplest (the chemical level—atoms and molecules) and ending with the most complex (the organism).
3. Describe the 10 principal organ systems.
4. Define metabolism, and contrast anabolism with catabolism.
5. Define homeostasis, and contrast negative and positive feedback mechanisms.
6. Describe the anatomical position of the human body.
7. Define and properly use the principal orientational terms employed in human anatomy.
8. Recognize sagittal, transverse, and frontal sections of the body and of body structures.
9. Define and locate the principal regions and cavities of the body.

STUDY QUESTIONS

Within each category, fill in the blanks with the correct response.

Introducing the Human Body

Adapted   Anatomy   Physiology   Shape   Structure

1. _____ is the science of body structure.

2. _____ is the science of body function.

3. Each structure of the body is precisely _____ for carrying out its specific function.

4. In the body, the size, _____, and _____ of each part are related to the job the part must perform.

I. THE BODY HAS SEVERAL LEVELS OF ORGANIZATION

Atoms	**Epithelial**	**Muscle**	**Organs**	**Body**	**Functions**
Nervous	**Tissue**	**Cells**	**Ion**	**Organ**	**Water**
Chemical	**Microscope**	**Organism**	**Connective**	**Molecules**	**Organelles**

1. The simplest level of organization in the body is the _____ level.

2. _____ are the basic units of matter.

3. An electrically charged atom is called a(n) _____.

4. Atoms combine chemically to form _____.

5. Two atoms of hydrogen combine with one atom of oxygen to form one molecule of

_____.

6. In living organisms, atoms and molecules associate in specific ways to form _____, the building blocks of the body.

7. Although cells vary in size and shape according to their function, most are so small that they can be seen

only with a(n) _____.

8. Each cell consists of specialized cell parts called _____.

9. The next highest level of organization after the cellular level is the _____ level.

10. A tissue is a group of closely associated cells specialized to perform particular _____.

11. The four main types of tissue in the body are _____, _____,

_____, and _____.

12. Various types of tissue are organized into _____, such as the brain, stomach, or heart.

13. A group of tissues and organs that work together to perform specific functions makes up a body system, or

_____ system.

14. Working together with great precision and complexity, the body systems make up the living

_____.

II. THE BODY IS COMPOSED OF INORGANIC COMPOUNDS AND ORGANIC COMPOUNDS

Amino	**Enzymes**	**Organic**	**Steroids**	**Carbohydrates**
Inorganic	**Proteins**	**DNA**	**Nucleic**	**RNA**

1. _____ compounds are relatively small, simple compounds such as water or salt, and are required for many cell activities such as transporting materials through cell membranes.

2. _____ compounds are large, complex compounds containing carbon. They are the chemical building blocks of the body.

3. _____ are sugars and starches; they are used by the body as fuel molecules and to store energy.

4. _____ are an important type of lipid that includes hormones such as the male and female sex hormones.

5. _____ are catalysts that regulate chemical reactions.

6. The kinds and amounts of _____ in a cell determine to a large extent what a cell looks like and how it functions.

7. Proteins are large, complex molecules composed of subunits called _____ acids.

8. Two very important _____ acids are DNA and RNA.

9. _____ makes up the genes, and contains the instructions for making all the proteins needed by the cell.

10. _____ is important in the process of manufacturing proteins.

III. THE BODY SYSTEMS WORK TOGETHER TO MAINTAIN LIFE

Digestive	**Endocrine**	**Integumentary**	**Muscular**	**Respiratory**

1. The _____ system covers and protects the body.

2. The _____ system regulates body chemistry and many body functions.

3. The _____ system exchanges gases between the blood and the external environment.

4. The _____ system ingests and digests foods and absorbs them into the blood.

5. The _____ system moves parts of the skeleton and aids movement of internal materials.

IV. METABOLISM IS ESSENTIAL TO MAINTENANCE, GROWTH, AND REPAIR OF THE BODY

Anabolism	**Building**	**Metabolism**	**Synthetic**	**ATP**	**Catabolism**
Nutrients	**Breaking down**	**Cellular respiration**	**Oxygen**		

1. The chemical processes that take place within the body are collectively called its

    _____.

2. Two phases of metabolism are _____ and _____.

3. Catabolism is the _____ phase of metabolism.

4. Cells obtain energy from food molecules by a complex series of catabolic chemical reactions called

    _____.

5. Nutrients are slowly broken down and the energy released is packaged within a special energy storage

    molecule called _____.

6. Cellular respiration requires both _____ and _____.

7. Anabolism is the _____ or _____ phase of metabolism.

V. HOMEOSTATIC MECHANISMS MAINTAIN AN APPROPRIATE INTERNAL ENVIRONMENT

Feedback system	**Negative feedback**	**Stressor**	**Homeostasis**
Positive	**Negative**	**Positive feedback**	

1. Metabolic activities are continuously occurring in every living cell and they must be carefully regulated to

    maintain _____—a consistent internal environment or steady state—for the body.

2. A _____ is a stimulus that disrupts homeostasis, causing stress within the body.

3. A _____ consists of a cycle of events in which information about a change is fed
    back into the system so that the regulator can control the process.

4. In a _____ system, the response of the regulator counteracts the inappropriate
    change, thereby restoring the steady state.

5. Most homeostatic mechanisms in the body are _____ feedback systems.

6. In a _____ system, the variation from the steady state sets off a series of events that
    intensify the changes.

7. The delivery of a baby is an example of a _____ feedback system.

VI. THE BODY HAS A BASIC PLAN

Bilateral   Cranium   Mirror   Vertebral column

1. The body consists of right and left halves that are _____ images; that is, the body has

    _____ symmetry.

2. Two structures that characterize humans as vertebrates are the _____, or brain case,

    and the backbone, or _____.

A. Directions in the Body Are Relative

Anatomical	**Closer**	**Lateral**	**Superficial**	**Anterior**	**Deep**	**Medial**
Superior	**Axis**	**Distal**	**Midline**	**Ventral**	**Caudal**	
Dorsal	**Posterior**	**Cephalic**	**Inferior**	**Proximal**		

1. In the _____ position, the body is erect, the eyes are looking forward, the arms are at the sides, and the palms and toes are directed forward.

2. The "north pole" of the human body is the top of the head, its most _____ point.

3. The "south pole" of the body is represented by the soles of the feet, its most _____ part.

4. The heart is superior to the stomach because it is _____ to the head.

5. The terms _____ and "cranial" are sometimes used instead of "superior."

6. The term _____ is sometimes used instead of the word "inferior."

7. The front (belly) surface of the body is _____ or _____.

8. The back surface of the body is _____ or _____.

9. The body _____ is an imaginary line extending from the center of the top of the head to the groin.

10. The main superior-inferior body axis is _____, going right through the midline of the body.

11. A structure is medial if it is closer to the _____ of the body than to another structure.

12. A structure is _____ if it is toward one side of the body.

13. When a structure is closer to the body midline or point of attachment to the trunk, it is described as

    _____.

14. _____ means farther from the midline or point of attachment to the trunk.

15. Structures located toward the surface of the body are _____.

16. Structures located farther inward are _____.

B. The Body Has Three Main Planes

Axes   **Midsagittal plane**   **Transverse plane**   **Frontal plane**   **Sagittal plane**

1. The body has three _____, each at right angles to the other two.

2. A _____ divides the body into right and left parts.

3. A _____ passes through the body axis and divides the body into two mirror-image halves.

4. A _____ divides the body into superior and inferior parts.

5. A _____ divides the body into anterior and posterior parts.

C. We Can Identify Specific Body Regions

Appendicular   **Cephalic**   **Cranial**   **Axial**   **Cervical**   **Torso**

1. The body may be subdivided into a(n) _____ portion, consisting of the head, neck, and trunk.

2. The _____ portion of the body consists of the limbs.

3. The _____ consists of the thorax, abdomen, and pelvis.

4. The _____ region refers to the head.

5. The _____ region refers to the neck.

6. The _____ region refers to the skull.

D.   The Body Has Two Main Cavities

Abdominopelvic   Diaphragm   Thoracic   Cavities   Dorsal   Ventral   Cranial   Pericardial   Vertebral

1.   The spaces within the body that contain the internal organs are called the body

_____.

2.   The principal body cavities are the _____ cavity and the

_____ cavity.

3.   The dorsal cavity is subdivided into the _____ cavity, which holds the brain, and the

_____ canal, which contains the spinal cord.

4.   The ventral cavity is subdivided into the _____, or chest cavity, and the

_____ cavity.

5.   The thoracic and abdominopelvic cavities are separated by a broad muscle, the

_____, which forms the floor of the thoracic cavity.

6.   The heart is surrounded by the _____ cavity.

E. It Is Important to View the Body as a Whole

Labeling Exercise

Please fill in the correct labels for Figure 1-1.

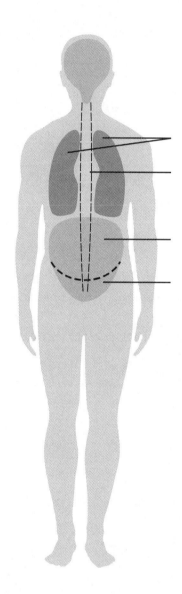

Figure 1-1

Labeling Exercise

Please fill in the correct labels for Figure 1-2.

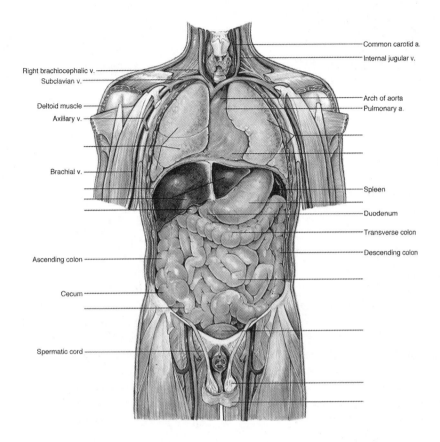

Figure 1-2

CHAPTER TEST

Select the correct response.

1. The study of anatomy is the
   a. science of body structure.
   b. science of body function.
   c. both a and b.
   d. science of insect classification.

2. The study of physiology is the
   a. science of body structure.
   b. science of body function.
   c. both a and b.
   d. science of mental illnesses.

3. An electrically charged atom is called a(n)
   a. proton.
   b. ion.
   c. electron.
   d. molecule.

4. Each cell consists of specialized cell parts called
   a. organs.
   b. protons.
   c. organelles.
   d. molecules.

5. The information and control center of the cell is the
   a. cytoplasm.
   b. neutron.
   c. nucleus.
   d. ribosome.

6. _____ are sugars and starches; they are used by the body as fuel molecules.
   a. Carbohydrates
   b. Fats
   c. Steroids
   d. Proteins

7. All of the chemical processes that take place within the body are collectively called its
   a. metabolism.
   b. mitosis.
   c. anabolism.
   d. chemicalism.

8. Steroids are an important group of _____ which include hormones; for example, male and female sex hormones.
   a. lipids
   b. carbohydrates
   c. glucose
   d. proteins

9. _____ are catalysts that regulate chemical reactions.
   a. Amino acids
   b. Enzymes
   c. Lipids
   d. Carbohydrates

10. Proteins are composed of subunits called
    a. amino acids.
    b. nucleic acids.
    c. carbohydrates.
    d. lipids.

11. _____ is a nucleic acid that makes up the genes (hereditary material).
    a. RNA
    b. DNA
    c. ERA
    d. ATP

12. Human cells obtain energy from food molecules through a complex series of chemical reactions called
    a. homeostasis.
    b. cellular respiration.
    c. anabolism.
    d. catabolic energy production.

13. Metabolic activities occur continuously in every living cell and they must be carefully regulated to maintain
    a. cellular respiration.
    b. positive feedback.
    c. homeostasis.
    d. metabolism.

14. When the body is erect with the eyes looking forward, the arms at the sides, and the palms and toes directed forward, it is said to be in the _____ position.
    a. standing
    b. front
    c. anatomical
    d. physiological

15. When the body is in the anatomical position, the brain is _____ to the heart.
    a. inferior
    b. superior
    c. superficial
    d. It depends on the individual.

16. The ____ plane divides the body into right and left parts.
    a. sagittal
    b. transverse
    c. frontal
    d. mirror

17. The dorsal cavity is subdivided into the _____ cavity, which holds the brain, and the _____ canal, which contains the spinal cord.
    a. ventral; cranial
    b. vertebral; spinal
    c. cranial; vertebral
    d. ventral; cranial

18. The ventral cavity is subdivided into the _____ cavity and the _____ cavity.
    a. thoracic; chest
    b. thoracic; abdominopelvic
    c. thoracic; diaphragm
    d. dorsal; ventral

Chapter

2

CELLS AND TISSUES

■ ■ ■

Outline

I. The cell contains specialized organelles that perform specific functions.
II. Materials move through the plasma membrane by both passive and active processes.
III. Cells divide by mitosis, forming genetically identical cells.

IV. Tissues are the fabric of the body.
   A. Epithelial tissue protects the body.
   B. Connective tissue joins body structures.
   C. Muscle tissue is specialized to contract.
   D. Nervous tissue controls muscles and glands.
V. Membranes cover or line body surfaces.

Learning Objectives

After you have studied this chapter, you should be able to:

1. Describe the general characteristics of cells.
2. Describe, locate, and list the functions of the principal organelles and label them on a diagram.
3. Explain how materials pass through cell membranes, distinguishing between passive and active processes.
4. Predict whether cells will swell or shrink under various osmotic conditions.

5. Describe the stages of a cell's life cycle, and summarize the significance of mitosis with respect to maintaining a constant chromosome number.
6. Define the term *tissue* and give the functions of the principal types of tissues.
7. Compare epithelial tissue with connective tissue.
8. Compare the three types of muscle tissue.
9. Identify the main types of membranes and contrast the main types of epithelial membranes.

STUDY QUESTIONS

Within each category, fill in the blanks with the correct response.

I. THE CELL CONTAINS SPECIALIZED ORGANELLES THAT PERFORM SPECIFIC FUNTIONS

Amino acids	DNA	Golgi complex	Nucleus	Ribosomes	Cells
Electron	Light	Organelles	Rough	Lysosomes	Ovum
Smooth	Chromosomes	Free radicals	Microscope	Plasma	Cilia
Functions	Mitochondria	Proteins	Cytoplasm	Genome	Nucleolus
Receptors	Cellular respiration	Endoplasmic reticulum			

1. _____ are the living building blocks of the body.

2. The _____ is one of the biologist's most important tools for studying the internal structure of cells.

3. Most cell structures were first identified with an ordinary _____ microscope.

4. The development of the _____ microscope enabled researchers to study the fine detail (ultrastructure) of cells and their parts.

5. The size and shape of a cell are related to the specific _____ it must perform.

6. The _____ is one of the largest cells in the human body.

7. The jellylike material of the cell is called _____.

8. _____ found in the cytoplasm are used to manufacture larger molecules such as proteins.

9. Scattered throughout the cell are specialized _____ (little organs) that perform different functions within the cell.

10. Every cell is surrounded by a thin membrane called the _____ membrane.

11. _____ project from the surface of the plasma membrane and receive chemical messages from endocrine glands or other types of cells.

12. The _____ is a large, round organelle that is the control center of the cell.

13. When a cell prepares to divide, the chromatin in the nucleus becomes more tightly coiled and condenses to

    form rod-shaped bodies called _____.

14. Genes, arranged in a specific linear order, are composed of the chemical compound

    _____.

15. The complete set of genes that make up the human genetic material is the human

    _____.

16. The _____ is a specialized region within the nucleus where ribosomes are assembled.

17. The _____ is a system of membranes that extends throughout the cytoplasm.

18. There are two types of endoplasmic reticulum: _____ and

    _____.

19. Rough endoplasmic reticulum has a granular appearance that results from the presence along its outer walls

    of organelles called _____.

20. Ribosomes function as factories in which _____ are manufactured.

21. The _____ is composed of layers of platelike membranes that give it the appearance of a stack of pancakes.

22. An important function of the Golgi complex is to produce _____.

23. Cells contain tiny power plants called _____.

24. Inside the mitochondria, fuel molecules are broken down and energy is released; this process is called

_____.

25. Mitochondria can affect health and aging by leaking electrons that form _____.

26. _____ are tiny hairlike organelles that project from the surfaces of many types of cells and help move materials outside the cell.

Labeling Exercise

Please fill in the correct labels for Figure 2-1.

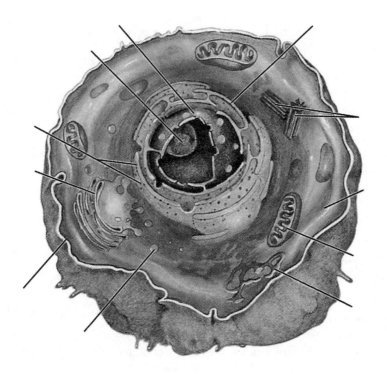

Figure 2-1

II. MATERIALS MOVE THROUGH THE PLASMA MEMBRANE

Active transport Filtration Permeable Diffusion Osmosis Phagocytosis

1. The plasma membrane is selectively _____.

2. _____ is the net movement of molecules or ions from a region of higher concentration to a region of lower concentration brought about by the energy of the molecules.

3. _____ is the diffusion of water molecules through a selectively permeable membrane from a region in which water molecules are more concentrated to a region in which they are less concentrated.

4. _____ is the passage of materials through membranes by mechanical pressure.

5. _____ requires cellular energy. In this process, the cell moves materials from a region of lower concentration to a region of higher concentration.

6. In _____, the cell ingests large, solid particles such as food or bacteria.

III. CELLS DIVIDE BY MITOSIS, FORMING GENETICALLY IDENTICAL CELLS

Anaphase Interphase Prophase Chromosomes Metaphase Telophase Five Mitosis Two

1. Before a cell divides to form two cells, the chromosomes are precisely duplicated, and the cell undergoes

    _____.

2. In mitosis, a complete set of _____ is distributed to each end of the parent cell.

3. The life cycle of the cell may be divided into _____ phases.

4. The cell spends most of its life in _____.

5. _____ is the first stage of mitosis.

6. During _____, the chromosomes are positioned along the equator of the cell.

7. During _____, chromatids separate and become independent chromosomes.

8. _____ begins with the arrival of a complete set of chromosomes at each end of the cell.

9. During telophase, the cell divides, forming _____ cells.

IV.   TISSUES ARE THE FABRIC OF THE BODY

Connective   Histology   Nervous   Epithelial   Muscle   Tissue

1.   A _____ is a group of closely associated cells that work together to carry out a specific function or group of functions.

2.   The four principal types of tissue that make up the body are _____,

_____, _____, and _____.

3.   The microscopic study of tissues is called _____.

A.   Epithelial Tissue Protects the Body

Absorb   Endocrine   Gland   Squamous   Columnar   Epithelial
Stratified   Cuboidal   Exocrine   Simple   Thyroid   Pseudostratified

1.   _____ tissue protects the body by covering all of its free surfaces and lining its cavities.

2.   In some parts of the body, epithelial tissue is specialized to _____ certain materials.

3.   _____ epithelial cells are thin, flattened cells shaped like pancakes or flagstones.

4.   _____ epithelial cells are short cylinders that from the side appear to cube-shaped, resembling dice.

5.   _____ epithelial cells look like columns or cylinders when viewed from the side.

6.   Epithelial tissue may be _____, composed of one layer of cells; or

_____, composed of two or more layers.

7.   _____ epithelium gives the illusion that the cells are layered because the cells are of different heights and their nuclei are at different levels in the tissue.

8.   A(n) _____ consists of one or more epithelial cells that produce and discharge a particular product.

9.   Two main types of glands are _____ and _____ glands.

10.   The _____ gland is an example of an endocrine gland.

B.   Connective Tissue Joins Body Structures

Adipose   **Fibroblasts**   **Macrophages**   **Collagen**   **Intercellular**   **Organ**
Elastic   **Join together**   **Reticular**   **Fibers**   **Loose**

1.   The main function of connective tissue is to _____ the other tissues of the body.

2.   Almost every _____ in the body has a supporting framework of connective tissue.

3.   Cells of connective tissue are usually separated by large amounts of _____ substance, which consists of threadlike microscopic _____ scattered throughout a thick gel or matrix.

4.   Three types of connective tissue fibers are _____, _____, and

_____.

5.   Two types of cells that are common in connective tissues are _____ and

_____.

6.   _____ connective tissue, or areolar tissue, joins body structures.

7.   _____ tissue stores fat and releases it when the body needs energy.

C.   Muscle Tissue Is Specialized to Contract

Contract   Involuntary   Skeletal   Smooth

1.   Muscle tissue is composed of cells specialized to _____.

2.   _____ muscle fibers have a striped, or striated, appearance; are attached to bone; and contract when stimulated by nerves.

3.   Cardiac muscle, found in the walls of the heart, is considered _____ because we do not generally make a conscious decision to contract it.

4.   _____ muscle is found in the walls of the digestive tract, uterus, blood vessels, and other internal organs. Its fibers are not striated and its control is involuntary.

D.   Nervous Tissue Controls Muscles and Glands

Axon   Dendrites   Neurons   Cell body   Glial   Sensory

1.   Nervous tissue consists of _____, cells that are specialized for transmitting nerve

impulses, and _____ cells that support and nourish the neurons.

2.   A typical neuron has a large _____, which contains the nucleus and from which two types of extensions project.

3.   _____ are specialized for receiving impulses, whereas the single

_____ conducts information away from the cell body.

4.   Neurons receive information from _____ receptors, structures that detect information about changes in the internal or external environment.

V.   MEMBRANES COVER OR LINE BODY SURFACES

Membranes   Parietal   Synovial   Mucous   Serous   Visceral

1.   _____ are sheets of tissue that cover or line body surfaces.

2.   A _____ membrane, or mucosa, lines body cavities that open to the outside of the body.

3.   A _____ membrane, or serosa, lines a body cavity that does not open to the outside of the body.

4.   A _____ membrane is a connective tissue membrane that lines a joint cavity.

5.   The part of the membrane that is attached to the wall of the cavity is the _____ membrane.

6.   The part of the membrane that covers the organs inside the cavity is the _____ membrane.

Labeling

Label each phase and describe what is happening in Figure 2-2.

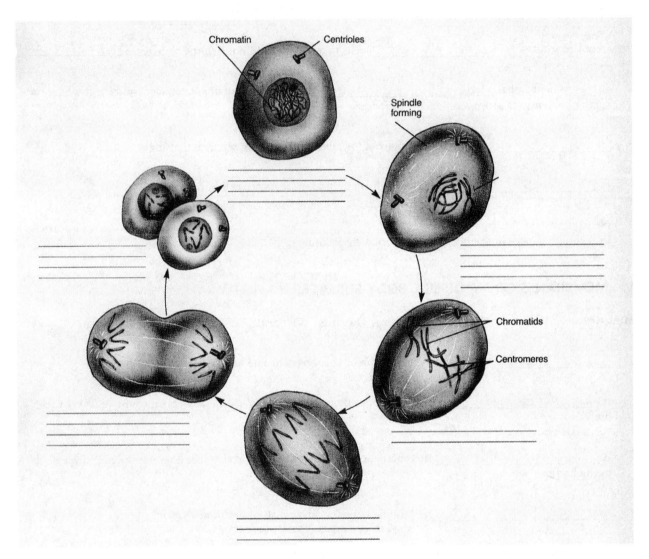

Figure 2-2

CHAPTER TEST

Select the correct response.

1. Cells associate to form
   a. atoms.
   b. molecules.
   c. tissues.
   d. ribosomes.

2. The _____ is one of the biologist's most important tools for studying the internal structure of cells.
   a. telescope
   b. binoculars
   c. stethoscope
   d. microscope

3. _____ cells look like tiny building blocks.
   a. Bone
   b. Epithelial
   c. Nerve
   d. Muscle

4. The jellylike material of the cell is called
   a. plasma membrane.
   b. cytoplasm.
   c. endoplasmic reticulum.
   d. ribosomes.

5. Every cell is surrounded by a thin membrane, the
   a. plasma membrane.
   b. cytoplasm.
   c. endoplasmic reticulum.
   d. ribosomes.

6. The _____ is a system of membranes that extends throughout the cytoplasm of many cells and through which materials can be transported from one part of the cell to another.
   a. plasma membrane
   b. mitochondria
   c. endoplasmic reticulum
   d. ribosomes

7. _____ function(s) as factories in the cell where proteins are manufactured.
   a. Mitochondria
   b. Endoplasmic reticulum
   c. Ribosomes
   d. Lysosomes

8. Looking like stacks of pancakes, the _____ is composed of layers of platelike membranes. This organelle functions as a protein processing and packaging plant.
   a. Golgi complex
   b. mitochondria
   c. endoplasmic reticulum
   d. ribosomes

9. _____ are little sacs that contain powerful digestive enzymes that destroy bacteria and other foreign matter.
   a. Golgi complex
   b. Mitochondria
   c. Endoplasmic reticulum
   d. Lysosomes

10. Cells contain tiny power plants called
    a. Golgi complex.
    b. mitochondria.
    c. endoplasmic reticulum.
    d. lysosomes.

11. The _____ is the control center of the cell.
    a. Golgi complex
    b. mitochondrion
    c. ribosome
    d. nucleus

12. The nucleus of a cell that is not in the process of dividing contains loosely coiled material called
    a. ATP.
    b. DNA.
    c. chromosomes.
    d. chromatin.

13. When a cell prepares to divide, the chromatin becomes more tightly coiled and condenses, forming rod-shaped bodies called
    a. ATP.
    b. DNA.
    c. chromosomes.
    d. lysosomes.

14. The _____ is a specialized region within the nucleus in which ribosomes are assembled.
    a. Golgi complex
    b. nucleolus
    c. mitochondria
    d. riboplex

15. _____ are tiny cells with long whiplike tails.
    a. Sperm
    b. Egg
    c. Nerve
    d. Muscle

16. _____ is the net movement of molecules or ions from a region of higher concentration to a region of lower concentration.
    a. Diffusion
    b. Osmosis
    c. Filtration
    d. Phagocytosis

17. _____ is the active transport of water molecules through a selectively permeable membrane from a region in which water molecules are more concentrated to a region in which they are less concentrated.
    a. Diffusion
    b. Osmosis
    c. Filtration
    d. Phagocytosis

18. _____ is the passage of materials through membranes by mechanical pressure.
    a. Diffusion
    b. Osmosis
    c. Filtration
    d. Active transport

19. _____ requires cellular energy for a cell to move material from a region of lower concentration to a region of higher concentration.
    a. Diffusion
    b. Osmosis
    c. Filtration
    d. Active transport

20. In _____, the cell ingests large, solid particles of food or bacteria.
    a. osmosis
    b. filtration
    c. active transport
    d. phagocytosis

21. In _____, a complete set of chromosomes moves to the opposite ends of the parent cell.
    a. mitosis
    b. interphase
    c. anaphase
    d. prophase

22. _____ can be considered a phase in the life cycle of the cell.
    a. Interphase
    b. Prophase
    c. Metaphase
    d. All of the above

23. _____ tissue protects the body by covering all of its free surfaces and lining its cavities.
    a. Epithelial
    b. Connective
    c. Muscle
    d. Nervous

24. _____ tissues join the other tissues of the body.
    a. Epithelial
    b. Connective
    c. Muscle
    d. Nervous

25. _____ tissue stores fat and releases it when the body needs energy. It also helps to shape and protect the body and provides insulation.
    a. Areolar
    b. Adipose
    c. Collagen
    d. Cardiac

26. A _____ membrane lines body cavities that open to the outside of the body.
    a. serous
    b. mucous
    c. visceral
    d. tympanic

Chapter

3

INTEGUMENTARY SYSTEM

■ ■ ■

Outline

I. The skin functions as a protective barrier.
II. The skin consists of epidermis and dermis.
   A. The epidermis continuously replaces itself.
   B. The dermis provides strength and elasticity.
   C. The subcutaneous layer attaches the skin to underlying tissues.

III. Sweat glands help maintain body temperature.
IV. Sebaceous glands lubricate the hair and skin.
V. Hair and nails are appendages of the skin.
VI. Melanin helps determine skin color.

Learning Objectives

After you have studied this chapter, you should be able to:

1. List six functions of the skin and explain how each is important in homeostasis.
2. Compare the structure and function of the epidermis with those of the dermis.
3. Describe the subcutaneous layer.

4. Describe the functions of sweat glands and sebaceous glands.
5. Describe the functions of hair and nails, and describe the structure of a hair.
6. Explain the function of melanin.

STUDY QUESTIONS

Within each category, fill in the blanks with the correct response.

I. THE SKIN FUNCTIONS AS A PROTECTIVE BARRIER

Fluid   Integumentary system   Sensory receptors   Vitamin D

1. Together with its glands, hair, and nails, the skin makes up the _____.

2. Located within the skin are _____ that detect touch, pressure, heat, cold, and pain.

3. The skin prevents loss of _____ and thereby prevents cells from drying out.

4. The skin contains a compound that is converted to _____ when it is exposed to the ultraviolet rays of the sun.

II. THE SKIN CONSISTS OF THE EPIDERMIS AND DERMIS

Dermis   Epidermis   Subcutaneous

1. The outer layer of the skin is called the _____.

2. The inner layer of the skin is called the _____.

3. Beneath the skin is an underlying _____ layer.

A. The Epidermis Continuously Replaces Itself

Deepest   Epithelial   Outer   Die   Keratin

1. The epidermis consists of stratified squamous _____ tissue.

2. The _____ cells of the epidermis continuously wear off.

3. New epidermal cells are constantly produced in the _____ sublayer of the epidermis.

4. _____, a tough, waterproofing protein, gives the skin mechanical strength and flexibility.

5. As epidermal cells move through the outer sublayer of epidermis, they _____.

B. The Dermis Provides Strength and Elasticity

Collagen   Glands   Temperature   Connective   Hair follicles   Fingerprints   Papillae

1. Dermis consists of dense _____ tissue composed mainly of collagen fibers.

2. _____ allows the skin to stretch and return to its normal form again.

3. Specialized skin structures such as _____ and _____ are found in the dermis.

4. The upper portion of the dermis has many small, fingerlike extensions called _____ that project into the epidermal tissue.

5. Extensive networks of capillaries in the papillae deliver oxygen and nutrients to the cells of the epidermis,

   and also function in _____ regulation.

6. _____ serve as friction ridges that help us hold onto the objects we grasp.

C. The Subcutaneous Layer Attaches the Skin to Underlying Tissues

Adipose   Muscles   Superficial fascia   Fat   Shock

1. The subcutaneous layer beneath the dermis is also called the _____.

2. The subcutaneous layer attaches the skin to the _____ and other tissues beneath.

3. The thick, fatty, subcutaneous layer helps protect the underlying organs from mechanical

   _____.

4. Fat stored within the _____ tissue can be mobilized and used as an energy source when adequate food is not available.

5. Distribution of _____ in the subcutaneous layer is largely responsible for characteristic male and female body shapes.

III. SWEAT GLANDS HELP MAINTAIN BODY TEMPERATURE

Armpits   Genital   Nitrogen   Body temperature   Heat
Sweat gland   Evaporation   Increase   Water

1. Each _____ is a tiny coiled tube found in the dermis or subcutaneous tissue.

2. About 3 million sweat glands in the skin help maintain _____.

3. Muscle movement and metabolic activity generate _____ and therefore

   _____ body temperature.

4. Because heat is required for _____, the body becomes cooler as sweat evaporates from the skin.

5. Sweat glands also excrete excess water and some _____ wastes from the body.

6. About 1 qt of _____ is excreted each day.

7. Certain sweat glands found in association with hairs are concentrated in a few specific areas of the body,

   such as _____ and _____ areas.

IV. SEBACEOUS GLANDS LUBRICATE THE HAIR AND SKIN

Acne   Pimple   Sebum   Ducts   Sebaceous glands

1. _____, also known as oil glands, are generally attached to hair follicles.

2. Sebaceous glands are connected to each hair follicle by little _____ through which they release their secretions.

3. Sebaceous glands secrete an oily substance called _____.

4. Sometimes the duct of a sebaceous gland ruptures, allowing sebum to spill into the dermis. The skin may

   become inflamed and a _____ may form.

5. At puberty, the stepped-up activity of sebaceous glands can sometimes lead to _____, a condition that is very common during adolescence.

V. HAIR AND NAILS ARE APPENDAGES OF THE SKIN

Capillaries Follicle Palms Shaft Contract Keratin Protective Smooth Dead Nails Root Soles

1. Hair serves a _____ function.

2. Hair is found on all skin surfaces except the _____ and the

   _____.

3. The part of the hair that is visible is called the _____.

4. The part of the hair that is below the skin surface is called the _____.

5. The root together with its epithelial and connective tissue coverings are collectively called the hair

   _____.

6. At the bottom of the hair follicle is a little mound of connective tissue containing

   _____ that deliver nutrients to the cells of the follicle.

7. Each hair consists of cells that manufacture _____.

8. The shaft of the hair consists of _____ cells and their products.

9. Tiny bundles of _____ muscle are associated with hair follicles.

10. Arrector pili muscles _____ in response to cold or fear, causing the hairs to stand up straight.

11. _____ help protect the ends of the fingers and the toes.

VI. MELANIN HELPS DETERMINE SKIN COLOR

Absorbs Carotene Lowest Sunburned Albino Color Melanin Ultraviolet Cancer Darker Sun

1. Scattered throughout the _____ layer of the epidermis are cells that produce pigment granules.

2. Pigment granules are composed of a type of protein called _____.

3. Melanin gives _____ to hair as well as to skin.

4. _____ is a yellowish pigment found with melanin in people of Asian descent.

5. A(n) _____ is a person of any race who has inherited the inability to produce pigment.

6. Melanin is an important protective screen against the _____.

7. Melanin _____ harmful ultraviolet rays.

8. Exposure to the sun stimulates an increase in the amount of melanin produced and causes the skin to become

_____.

9. A dark tan is actually a sign that the skin has been exposed to too much _____ radiation.

10. When the melanin is not able to absorb all of the ultraviolet rays, the skin becomes inflamed, or

_____.

11. Over a period of years, excessive exposure to the sun can cause wrinkling of the skin, and sometimes skin

_____.

Labeling Exercise

Please fill in the correct labels for Figure 3-1.

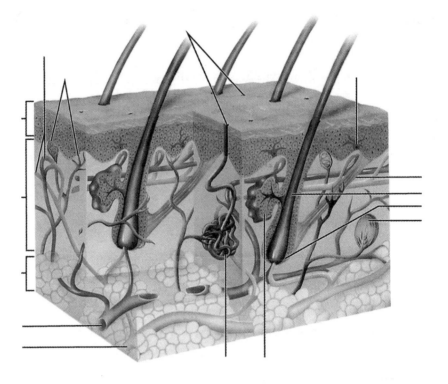

Figure 3-1

CHAPTER TEST

Select the correct response.

1. The skin, with its glands, hair, and nails, makes up the
   a. dermal system.
   b. epidermal system.
   c. integumentary system.
   d. endocrine system.

2. Oxygen and nutrients are delivered to cells of the epidermis by
   a. arterioles in the superficial fascia.
   b. capillaries in the dermal papillae.
   c. capillaries in the upper sublayer of the epidermis.
   d. hair follicle sinuses.

3. The skin is responsible for
   a. protecting the body against injury.
   b. preventing internal body cells from drying out.
   c. maintaining body temperature.
   d. all of the above.

4. The skin contains a compound that is converted to _____ when the skin is exposed to the ultraviolet rays of the sun.
   a. vitamin A
   b. vitamin C
   c. vitamin D
   d. para-aminobenzoic acid (PABA)

5. The outer layer of the skin is called the
   a. epidermis.
   b. dermis.
   c. subcutaneous layer.
   d. adipose layer.

6. The inner layer of the skin is called the
   a. epidermis.
   b. dermis.
   c. subcutaneous layer.
   d. adipose layer.

7. The epidermis consists of stratified squamous _____ tissue.
   a. nerve
   b. connective
   c. epithelial
   d. muscle

8. The tough, waterproofing protein that fills most of each skin cell is called
   a. melanin.
   b. keratin.
   c. hydrotin.
   d. carotene.

9. The dermis consists of dense _____ tissue composed mainly of collagen fibers.
   a. nerve
   b. connective
   c. epithelial
   d. muscle

10. Collagen is largely responsible for the _____ of the skin.
    a. color
    b. elasticity
    c. cooling
    d. tanning ability

11. The subcutaneous layer beneath the dermis consists of loose _____ tissue.
    a. nerve
    b. connective
    c. epithelial
    d. muscle

12. Fat stored within the _____ tissue can be mobilized and used as an energy source when adequate food is not available.
    a. adipose
    b. epithelial
    c. nerve
    d. reserve

13. Sweat glands are tiny coiled tubes in the
    a. epidermis.
    b. dermis.
    c. exoskeleton.
    d. out-skin.

14. There are approximately _____ sweat glands in the skin that help maintain body temperature.
    a. 3 million
    b. 7 hundred
    c. 20 thousand
    d. too many to count

15. Hair is found on all skin surfaces except the
    a. palms and soles.
    b. palms and fingers.
    c. fingers and soles.
    d. toes and fingers.

16. _____ is caused by the contraction of the arrector pili muscles.
    a. Sweat
    b. Body odor
    c. Gooseflesh
    d. Keratin

17. Nails appear pink because of underlying
    a. carotene.
    b. veins.
    c. arteries.
    d. capillaries.

18. In dark-skinned individuals, the pigment cells are more active and produce more
    a. blood.
    b. ultraviolet rays.
    c. carotene.
    d. melanin.

19. People who sunbathe are more prone to _____ than are people who do not stay out in the sun very long.
    a. wrinkles
    b. skin cancer
    c. sunburn
    d. all of the above

CROSSWORD PUZZLE FOR CHAPTERS 1, 2, AND 3

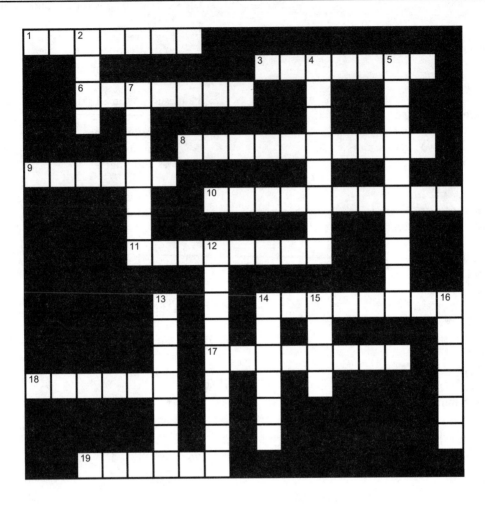

Across

1. Pertains to the skull
3. Science of body structure
6. Movement of water across a cell membrane
8. Tissue that lines body cavities
9. Cell that transmits nerve impulses
10. Science of body function
11. Higher in the body
14. Closer to the body midline
17. Fibrous protein that is the main support of many connective tissues
18. Closer to the body midline
19. Group of cells aggregated to perform a function

Down

2. Smallest unit of an element that retains the chemical properties of that element
4. Ventral
5. Chemical processes that occur within the body
7. Division of the cell nucleus
12. Glands that secrete hormones
13. Control center of a cell
14. The bony ring that supports the lower portion of trunk
15. Relating to the mouth
16. Region of the lower back

Chapter

THE SKELETAL SYSTEM

■ ■ ■

Outline

I. The skeletal system supports and protects the body.
II. A typical long bone consists of a shaft with flared ends.
III. Two types of bone tissue are compact and spongy bone.
IV. Bone develops by replacing existing connective tissue.
V. The bones of the skeleton are grouped in two divisions.
VI. The axial skeleton consists of 80 bones.
  A. The skull is the bony framework of the head.
  B. The vertebral column supports the body.
  C. The thoracic cage protects the organs of the chest.

VII. The appendicular skeleton consists of 126 bones.
  A. The pectoral girdle attaches the upper extremities (limbs) to the axial skeleton.
  B. The bones of the upper extremity (limb) are located in the arm, forearm, wrist, and hand.
  C. The pelvic girdle supports the lower limbs.
  D. The bones of the lower extremity (limb) are located in the thigh, knee, leg, ankle, and foot.
VIII. Joints are junctions between bones.
  A. Joints can be classified according to the degree of movement they permit.
  B. A diarthrosis is surrounded by a joint capsule.

Learning Objectives

After you have studied this chapter, you should be able to:

1. List five functions of the skeletal system.
2. Label a diagram of a long bone and describe the microscopic structure of a bone.
3. Contrast endochondral with intramembranous bone development.
4. Describe the role of osteoblasts and osteoclasts in bone production and remodeling.

5. List and describe the bones of the axial skeleton and identify each on a diagram or skeleton.
6. List and describe the bones of the appendicular skeleton and identify each on a diagram or skeleton.
7. Compare the main types of joints.
8. Describe the structure and functions of a diarthrosis.

STUDY QUESTIONS

Within each category, fill in the blanks with the correct response.

I. THE SKELETAL SYSTEM SUPPORTS AND PROTECTS THE BODY

Bones Marrow Tendons Interaction Protect Ligaments Support

1. The skeletal system functions to _____ the body by serving as a bony framework for

   the other tissues and organs and to _____ delicate vital organs.

2. _____ serve as levers that transmit muscular forces.

3. Muscles are attached to bones by bands of connective tissue called _____.

4. Bones are held together at the joints by bands of connective tissue called _____.

5. The _____ within some bones produces blood cells.

6. The _____ of bones and muscles also makes breathing possible.

II. A TYPICAL LONG BONE CONSISTS OF A SHAFT WITH FLARED ENDS

Bone Epiphyseal Metaphysis Diaphysis Epiphysis Periosteum Endosteum Hyaline Yellow

1. The main shaft of a long bone is called its _____.

2. The _____ is the expanded end of a long bone.

3. In children, a disc of cartilage called the _____ is found between the epiphysis and
   the diaphysis.

4. The metaphyses are growth centers that disappear at maturity, becoming vague

   _____ lines.

5. At its joint surfaces, the outer layer of a bone consists of a thin layer of _____
   cartilage, the articular cartilage.

6. Each long bone is covered by the _____, a layer of specialized connective tissue.

7. The inner layer of the periosteum contains cells that produce _____.

8. Within the long bone, there is a central marrow cavity filled with a fatty connective tissue called

   _____ bone marrow.

9. The marrow cavity of the long bone is lined with a thin layer of cells called the

   _____.

III. TWO TYPES OF BONE TISSUE ARE COMPACT AND SPONGY BONE

Bone marrow	**Epiphyses**	**Osteons**	**Yellow**	**Canaliculi**
Haversian canals	**Red**	**Compact**	**Lacunae**	**Spindle**
Dense	**Osteocytes**	**Spongy**		

1. Two types of bone tissue are _____ bone and _____ bone.

2. Compact bone, which is very _____ and hard, is found near the surfaces of the bone where great strength is needed.

3. Compact bone consists of interlocking, _____-shaped units called

   _____, or haversian systems.

4. Within an osteon, _____ (the mature bone cells) are found in small cavities called

   _____.

5. Lacunae are arranged in concentric circles around central _____.

6. Threadlike extensions of the cytoplasm of the osteocytes extend through narrow channels called

   _____. These cellular extensions connect the osteocytes.

7. Spongy bone is found within the _____ and makes up the inner part of the wall of the diaphysis.

8. The spaces within the spongy bone are filled with _____.

9. _____ marrow found in certain bones produces blood cells, while

   _____ marrow consists mainly of fat cells.

IV. BONE DEVELOPS BY REPLACING EXISTING CONNECTIVE TISSUE

Bones	**Ossification**	**Resorption**	**Endochondral**	**Intramembranous**
Osteoblasts	**Shape**	**Enzymes**	**Lacunae**	**Osteoclasts**
Tissue	**Fetal**	**Marrow**	**Osteocytes**	**Hydroxyapatite**

1. Bone formation is called _____.

2. During _____ development, bones form in two ways.

3. The long bones develop from cartilage models, a process called _____ bone development.

4. The flat bones of the skull develop from a noncartilage connective tissue scaffold; this is called

   _____ bone development.

5. _____ are cells that produce bone.

6. A complex calcium phosphate called _____ is present in tissue fluid.

7. As the bone matrix forms around the osteoblasts, they become isolated within small spaces called

   _____.

8. When osteoblasts become embedded in the bone matrix, they are called _____.

9. _____ are the cells that break down bone, a process called bone

   _____.

10. Osteoclasts are very large cells that secrete _____, which digest bone.

11. Osteoclasts and osteoblasts work side by side to _____ bones and form the precise grain needed.

12. As muscles develop in response to physical activity, the _____ to which they are attached thicken and become stronger.

13. As bones grow, bone _____ must be removed from the interior, especially from the

    walls of the _____ cavity. This process keeps bones from becoming too heavy.

Labeling Exercise

Please fill in the correct labels for Figure 4-1.

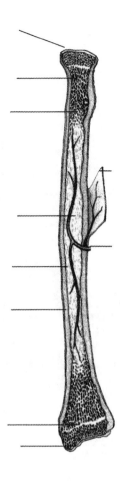

Figure 4-1

V. THE BONES OF THE SKELETON ARE GROUPED IN TWO DIVISIONS

206   Axial   Appendicular

1. The human skeleton consists of _____ named bones.

2. The _____ skeleton consists of the skull, vertebral column, ribs, and sternum.

3. The _____ skeleton consists of the upper and lower limbs, shoulder girdle, and pelvic girdle (with the exception of the sacrum).

Labeling Exercise

Please fill in the correct labels for Figure 4-2.

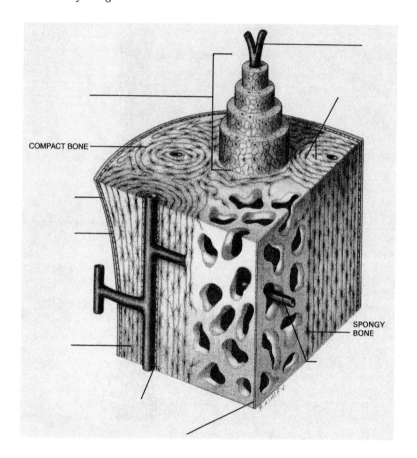

COMPACT BONE

SPONGY BONE

Figure 4-2

VI. THE AXIAL SKELETON CONSISTS OF 80 BONES

Atlas   Parietal   Sternum   Mandible   Ribs   Temporomandibular

1. The two _____ bones form much of the walls and roof of the cranium.

2. The _____ is the lower jaw bone. It joins with the temporal bone on each side to

   form the _____ joints.

3. The _____ is also known as the breast bone.

4. The _____ is the first cervical vertebra.

5. The _____ protect the organs of the thoracic cavity, and form part of the thoracic
   cage.

A.   The Skull Is the Bony Framework of the Head

Anterior	Fontanelles	Paranasal	Soft spots	Coronal	Frontal	Sagittal suture
Sutures	Cranium	Sinuses	Face	Middle	Sinusitis	Lambdoid suture

1. The skull, the bony framework of the head, is divided into the 8 bones of the _____
    and the 14 bones that make up the _____.

2. Contained within the head are six very small bones in the _____ ears.

3. Most of the bones of the skull are joined by the immovable joints called _____.

4. The _____ is the joint between the two parietal bones.

5. The coronal suture joins the parietal bones to the _____ bone.

6. The _____ is the joint between the parietal bones and the occipital bone.

7. In babies, six joints called _____ occur at the angles of the parietal bone.

8. The largest fontanelle is the _____ fontanelle, and it is found at the junction of the

    sagittal and _____ sutures.

9. The fontanelles, popularly called _____, permit the baby's head to be compressed
    slightly as it passes through the bony pelvis during birth.

10. _____ are air spaces lined with mucous membrane; they are found in some of the
    cranial bones.

11. Four pairs of sinuses, the _____ sinuses, are continuous with the nose and throat.

12. Sometimes the mucous membranes of the sinuses become swollen and inflamed and produce the condition

    called _____.

B.   The Vertebral Column Supports the Body

24	Discs	Sacrum	Cervical	Spine	Coccygeal
Fused	Thoracic	Coccyx	Intervertebral discs	Vertebral foramen	Five

1. The vertebral column, or _____, supports the body and bears its weight.

2. The vertebral column consists of _____ vertebrae.

3. The two fused bones of the vertebral column are the _____ and the

    _____.

4. The regions of the vertebral column are the _____, which consists of seven

   vertebrae; the _____, which consists of 12 vertebrae; the lumbar, which consists of

   _____ vertebrae; the sacral, which consists of five _____

   vertebrae; and the _____, which consists of 3-5 fused vertebrae.

5. The vertebrae articulate with each other by means of synovial joints and by means of

   _____ composed of cartilage.

6. The intervertebral _____ are tiny pads that act as shock absorbers.

7. The body and neural arch of the vertebra enclose a large opening called the _____.

Labeling Exercise

Please fill in the correct labels for Figure 4-3.

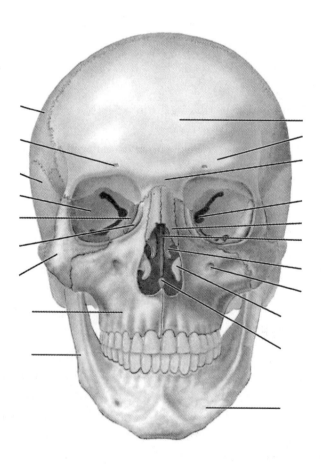

Figure 4-3

Labeling Exercise

Please fill in the correct labels for Figure 4-4.

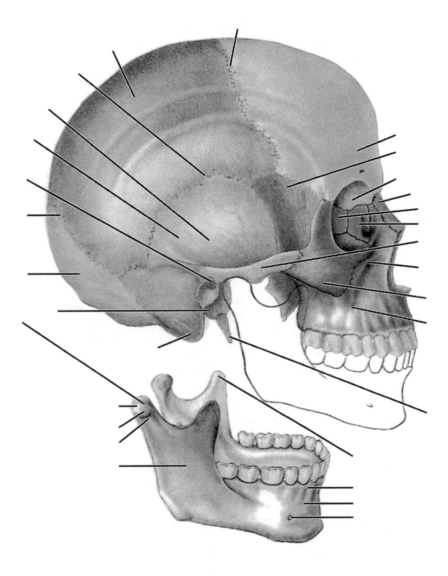

Figure 4-4

Labeling Exercise

Please fill in the correct labels for Figure 4-5.

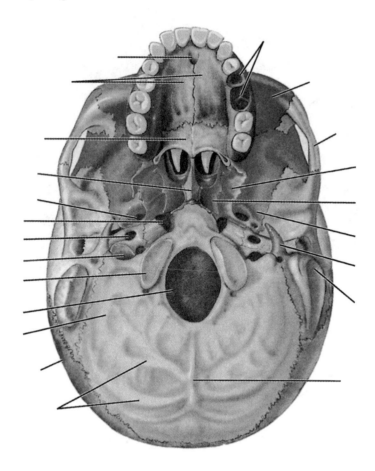

Figure 4-5

C. The Thoracic Cage Protects the Organs of the Chest

12 Rib Thoracic Pectoral Sternum

1. The thoracic cage, or _____ cage, protects the internal organs of the chest, including the heart and lungs.

2. The thoracic cage provides support for the bones of the _____ girdle and upper limbs.

3. The thoracic cage is a bony cage formed by the _____ , the

_____ vertebrae, and _____ pairs of ribs.

Labeling Exercise

Please fill in the correct labels for Figure 4-6.

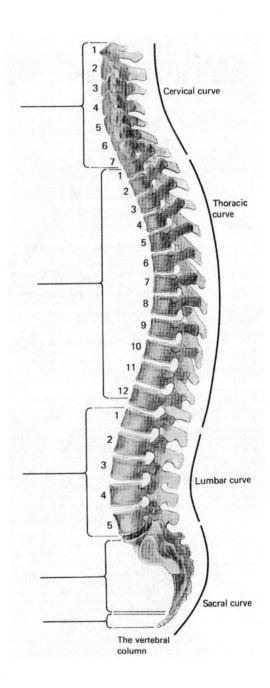

Figure 4-6

Labeling Exercise

Please fill in the correct labels for Figure 4-7.

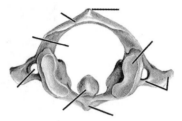

(a) Atlas seen from above

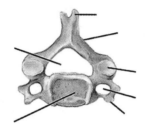

(b) Cervical vertebra seen from above

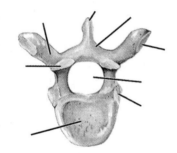

(c) Thoracic vertebra seen from above

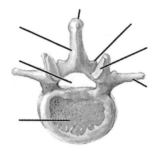

(d) Lumbar vertebra seen from above

Figure 4-7

VII.   THE APPENDICULAR SKELETON

Appendicular   Humerus   Patella   Pelvic   Femur   Metacarpals   Pectoral

1. The _____ skeleton consists of the bones of the upper and lower limbs, plus the

    bones making up the _____ girdle, and the _____ girdle
    (with the exception of the sacrum).

2. The _____ is the largest bone in the body.

3. The _____ is also known as the kneecap.

4. The _____ is the upper arm bone.

5. The heads of the _____ are the knuckles.

A.   The Pectoral Girdle Attaches the Upper Extremities (Limbs) to the Axial Skeleton

Clavicle   Glenoid   Spine   Sternum

1. Each pectoral girdle consists of a scapula and a(n) _____ .

2. The pectoral girdles articulate with the _____ but not with the vertebral column.

3. The _____ fossa is the socket that receives the head of the humerus.

4. The _____ of the scapula is a sharp ridge that runs diagonally across the posterior
    surface.

B.   Bones of the Upper Extremity (Limb) Are Located in the Arm, Forearm, Wrist, and Hand

30   Humerus   Phalanges   Ulna   Carpal   Metacarpal   Radius

1. Each upper limb consists of _____ bones.

2. The _____ is the bone in the upper arm.

3. The _____ and the _____ are the bones of the forearm.

4. The _____ bones form the wrist.

5. The _____ bones are in the palm of the hand.

6. The _____ are the bones of the fingers.

Labeling Exercise

Please fill in the correct labels for Figure 4-8.

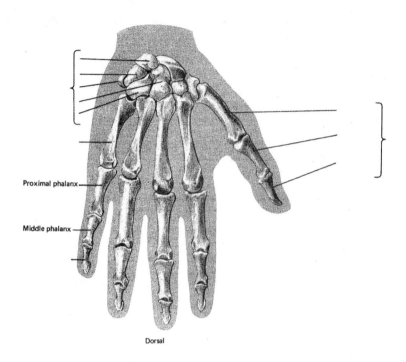

Proximal phalanx

Middle phalanx

Dorsal

Figure 4-8

C.   The Pelvic Girdle Supports the Lower Limbs

Coccyx Ischium Sacrum Coxal Pelvic Symphysis Ilium Pubis

1.   The _____ girdle is a broad basin of bone that encloses the pelvic cavity.

2.   The hip bones are called _____ bones.

3.   The coxal bones together with the _____ and _____ form the pelvic girdle.

4.   Each coxal bone is formed from the fusion of three bones. The largest of the three is the

     _____.

5.   The most posterior part of the coxal bone is the _____.

6.   The anterior part of the coxal bone is the _____.

7.   The joint where the coxal bones come together is called the pubic _____.

Labeling Exercise

Please fill in the correct labels for Figure 4-9.

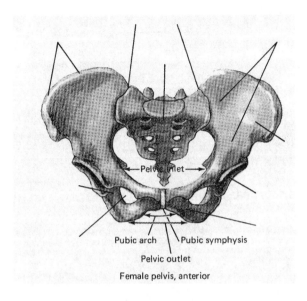

Pelvic inlet

Pubic arch   Pubic symphysis

Pelvic outlet

Female pelvis, anterior

Figure 4-9

D.   Bones of the Lower Extremity (Limb) Are Located in the Thigh, Knee, Leg, Ankle, and Foot

30   Metatarsal   Tarsal   Femur   Patella   Tibia   Fibula   Phalanges

1.   The lower limb consists of _____ bones.

2.   The _____ is the bone in the upper leg (thigh).

3.   The _____ is the kneecap.

4.   The _____ and _____ make up the bones of the lower leg.

5.   The bones of the heel and back part of the foot are called _____ bones.

6.   The _____ bones make up the main part of the foot.

7.   The _____ are the bones in the toes.

Labeling Exercise

Please fill in the correct labels for Figure 4-10.

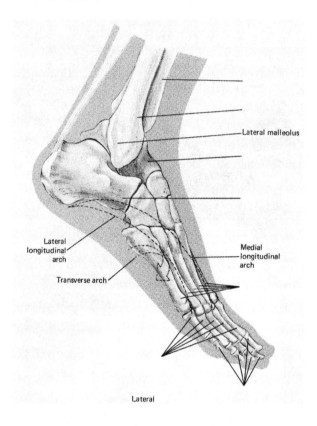

Lateral malleolus

Lateral
longitudinal
arch

Medial
longitudinal
arch

Transverse arch

Lateral

Figure 4-10

VIII.   JOINTS ARE JUNCTIONS BETWEEN BONES

Articulation   Ball-and-socket   Hinge   Pivot

1.   A joint, or _____, is the point of contact between two bones.

2.   The hip and shoulder joints are examples of _____ joints.

3.   The elbow and knee are _____ joints.

4.   The type of joint that allows the bones to rotate is a _____ joint.

A.   Joints Can Be Classified According to the Degree of Movement They Permit

Amphiarthroses   Fibrous   Synarthroses   Cartilage   Intervertebral   Synovial   Diarthroses   Skull   Three

1.   Joints can be classified into _____ main groups.

2. _____ are joints that do not permit movement. They connect bones by means of

   _____ connective tissue.

3. The sutures that join the _____ bones are synarthroses.

4. _____ permit slight movement, and are joined by _____ .

5. The _____ joints of the vertebral column are examples of amphiarthroses.

6. _____ , or synovial joints, are freely movable joints.

7. The six types of _____ joints are gliding, condyloid, saddle, pivot, hinge, and ball-
   and-socket.

B.   A Diarthrosis Is Surrounded by a Joint Capsule

Bursae   Hyaline   Ligaments   Bursitis   Joint   Synovial

1. The ends of the bones forming a diarthrodial joint are covered with _____ cartilage
   that lacks any sort of covering membrane.

2. The joint is surrounded by a connective tissue capsule, the _____ capsule.

3. The joint capsule is generally reinforced with _____ , bands of fibrous connective
   tissue that connect the bones and limit movement at the joint.

4. The joint capsule is lined with a membrane that secretes a lubricating fluid called

   _____ fluid.

5. Fluid-filled sacs called _____ are located between bone and tendons.

6. Inflammation of a bursa is a painful condition known as _____ .

CHAPTER TEST

Select the correct response.

1. The sternum and ribs protect the
    a. heart.
    b. stomach.
    c. lungs.
    d. both a and c.

2. The _____ within some bones produces blood cells.
    a. osteon
    b. lacuna
    c. marrow
    d. cartilage

3. The main shaft of the long bone is called its
    a. epiphyses.
    b. diaphysis.
    c. endosteum.
    d. periosteum.

4. The thin cellular layer that lines the marrow cavity is the
    a. pericardium.
    b. periosteum.
    c. endosteum.
    d. diaphysis.

5. Osteocytes are found in small cavities (within the osteon) called
    a. lacunae.
    b. canaliculi.
    c. osteoclasts.
    d. osteoblasts.

6. Spongy bone is found within the
    a. canaliculi.
    b. epiphyses.
    c. lacunae.
    d. haversian canals.

7. When osteoblasts become embedded in the bone matrix, they are called
    a. matrix marrow.
    b. lacunae.
    c. osteocytes.
    d. osteoclasts.

8. _____ work side by side to shape bones and form the precise grain needed in the finished bone.
    a. Lacunae and haversian canals
    b. Apatite and marrow
    c. Osteoblasts and matrix
    d. Osteoblasts and osteoclasts

9. The axial skeleton consists of the vertebral column, ribs, sternum, and
    a. upper and lower extremities.
    b. pectoral girdle.
    c. pelvic girdle.
    d. skull.

10. The appendicular skeleton consists of the upper and lower limbs, shoulder girdle, and
    a. pelvic girdle.
    b. skull.
    c. ribs.
    d. sternum.

11. The _____ suture is the joint between the parietal bones and the occipital bone.
    a. sagittal
    b. parietal
    c. coronal
    d. lambdoid

12. The paranasal sinuses are located in the
    a. frontal bone.
    b. maxillary bone.
    c. sphenoid bone.
    d. all of the above.

13. The regions of the vertebral column are the cervical, thoracic, lumbar, coccygeal, and
    a. sacral.
    b. centrum.
    c. lamina.
    d. discs.

14. Vertebrae articulate with each other by means of _____ joints.
    a. inflexible
    b. synovial
    c. sacral
    d. thoracic

15. The thoracic cage protects the internal organs of the
    a. reproductive system.
    b. brain.
    c. chest.
    d. all of the above.

16. The thoracic cage contains _____ pairs of ribs.
    a. 24
    b. 6
    c. 12
    d. It depends on the individual.

17. The pectoral girdle attaches the upper limbs to the _____ skeleton.
    a. appendicular
    b. sacral
    c. external
    d. axial

18. Each pectoral girdle consists of a clavicle and a
    s. scalpel.
    b. scapula.
    c. sternum.
    d. pubis.

19. The upper extremity consists of the humerus, ulna, carpals, metacarpals, phalanges, and
    a. tibia.
    b. femur.
    c. sternum.
    d. radius.

20. The pelvic girdle is a broad basin of bone that encloses the _____ cavity.
    a. pelvic
    b. chest
    c. pubic
    d. ischial

21. Two coxal bones together with the sacrum and coccyx form the
    a. pelvic girdle.
    b. pectoral girdle.
    c. ischium.
    d. trunk.

22. The sutures that join skull bones together are an example of
    a. synarthroses.
    b. amphiarthroses.
    c. diarthroses.
    d. synovial joints.

23. The painful condition known as bursitis is a result of
    a. lack of bursae.
    b. too many bursae.
    c. inflammation of a bursa.
    d. the bursting of a bursa.

24. Which of the following joints is considered a ball-and-socket joint?
    a. elbow
    b. hip
    c. carpometacarpal
    d. atlantoaxial

Labeling Exercise

Please fill in the correct labels for Figure 4-11.

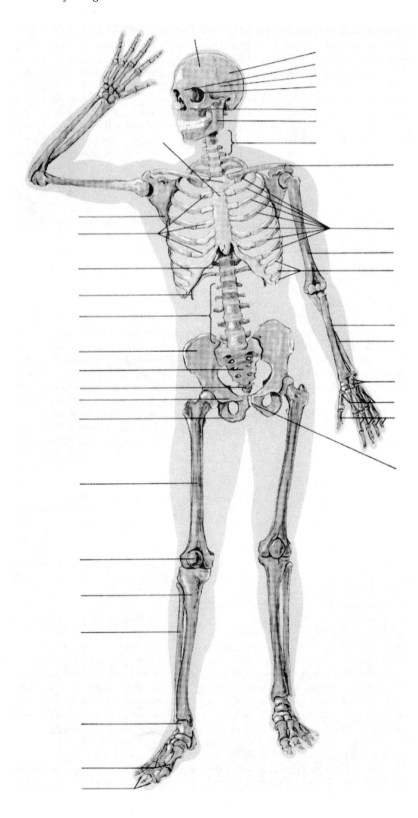

Figure 4-11

Chapter

THE MUSCULAR SYSTEM

■ ■ ■

Outline

Introduction
I. Skeletal muscle is composed of hundreds of muscle fibers.
II. Muscle fibers are specialized for contraction.
    A. Contraction occurs when actin and myosin filaments slide past each other.
    B. Muscle contraction requires energy.
C. Muscle tone is a state of partial contraction.
D. Two types of muscle contraction are isotonic and isometric.
III. Muscles work antagonistically to one another.
IV. We can study muscles in functional groups.

Learning Objectives

After you have studied this chapter, you should be able to:

1. Describe the structure of a skeletal muscle.
2. Relate the structure of a muscle fiber to its function.
3. List, in sequence, the events that occur during muscle contraction.
4. Compare the roles of glycogen, creatine phosphate, and ATP in providing energy for muscle contraction.
5. Define muscle tone and explain why muscle tone is important.
6. Distinguish between isotonic and isometric contraction.
7. Explain how muscles work antagonistically to one another.
8. Locate and give the actions of the principal muscles as indicated in Table 5-1 in the accompanying textbook.

STUDY QUESTIONS

Within each category, fill in the blanks with the correct response.

INTRODUCTION

Cardiac   Skeletal   Voluntary   Muscles   Smooth

1. All body movements depend on the action of _____.

2. The three types of muscles are _____, _____, and

   _____.

3. Skeletal muscles are the _____ muscles attached to bones.

I. SKELETAL MUSCLE IS COMPOSED OF HUNDREDS OF MUSCLE FIBERS

Endomysium Fascicles Perimysium Epimysium Fibers Tendons

1. Muscle cells are referred to as muscle _____.

2. Each muscle is surrounded by a covering of connective tissue called the _____.

3. The muscle fibers are arranged in bundles called _____.

4. Each fascicle is wrapped by connective tissue known as _____.

5. Individual muscle fibers are surrounded by a connective tissue covering called the

   _____.

6. Extensions of epimysium form tough cords of connective tissue called _____, which anchor muscles to bones.

II. MUSCLE FIBERS ARE SPECIALIZED FOR CONTRACTION

Actin Filaments Mitochondria Sarcomeres Contractile Myofibrils Myosin Transverse

1. Each muscle fiber is a spindle-shaped cell with several nuclei and numerous _____ that provide energy for muscle contraction.

2. The plasma membrane has many inward extensions that form a set of _____ tubules.

3. Each muscle fiber is almost filled with threadlike structures called _____ that run lengthwise through the muscle fiber.

4. Myofibrils are composed of smaller structures called _____ that are made of protein threads.

5. The thick filaments consisting mainly of the protein myosin are called _____ filaments.

6. The thin filaments consisting of the protein actin are called _____ filaments.

7. Myosin and actin are _____ proteins, which means that they are capable of shortening.

8. Myosin and actin filaments are organized into repeating units called _____, the basic units of muscle contraction.

A.   Contraction Occurs When Actin and Myosin Filaments Slide Past Each Other

Acetylcholine	Bridges	Motor	Calcium	Neuromuscular	Acetylcholinesterase
Action	Fibers	Synaptic	Bones	Impulses	

1.   Body movement occurs when muscles pull on _____ .

2.   A muscle contracts when its _____ contract.

3.   A(n) _____ nerve is a nerve that controls muscle contraction.

4.   Motor neurons (nerve cells) that make up a motor nerve transmit _____ to muscle fibers.

5.   The junction of a nerve and muscle fiber is called a(n) _____ junction.

6.   A motor neuron releases the neurotransmitter _____ .

7.   Acetylcholine is released into the _____ cleft between the motor neuron and muscle fiber.

8.   Depolarization may cause an electrical impulse, or _____ potential, to be generated in a muscle fiber.

9.   Excess acetylcholine is broken down by an enzyme called _____ .

10.   Depolarization of the T tubules opens calcium channels in the endoplasmic reticulum causing the release of

stored _____ .

11.   Energized myosin binds to the active sites on the actin filament, forming cross _____ that link the myosin and actin filaments.

B.   Muscle Contraction Requires Energy

ATP   Glucose   Oxygen debt   Creatine phosphate   Lactic acid   Fuel   Muscle fatigue

1.   The immediate source of energy for muscle contraction comes from the energy storage molecule,

_____ .

2.   In addition to ATP, muscle cells also have an energy storage compound called _____ .

3.   The energy for making creatine phosphate and ATP comes from _____ molecules.

4.   _____ , a simple sugar, is stored in muscle cells in the form of a large molecule called glycogen.

5. The depletion of ATP results in weaker contractions and _____.

6. A waste product called _____ is produced during anaerobic metabolism of glucose.

7. During muscle exertion, a(n) _____ may develop.

C. Muscle Tone Is a State of Partial Contraction

Motor nerve   Muscle tone   Posture   Unconscious

1. Even when they are not moving, muscles are in a state of partial contraction called

   _____.

2. Muscle tone is a(n) _____ process that helps keep muscles prepared for action.

3. Muscle tone is also responsible for helping the muscles of the abdominal wall hold the internal organs in place and is important in maintaining _____.

4. When the _____ to a muscle is cut, the muscle becomes limp, or flaccid.

D. Two Types of Muscle Contraction Are Isotonic and Isometric

Isometric   Isotonic

1. _____ contraction occurs when muscles shorten and thicken.

2. _____ contraction occurs when muscle length does not appreciably change but muscle tension increases.

III. MUSCLES WORK ANTAGONISTICALLY TO ONE ANOTHER

Agonist   Fixators   Synergists   Antagonist   Insertion   Tendons   Articulates   Origin

1. Skeletal muscles produce movements by pulling on _____, which in turn pull on bones.

2. When a muscle contracts, it draws one bone toward or away from the bone with which it

   _____.

3. The attachment of a muscle to a less movable bone is called its _____.

4. The attachment of a muscle to a more movable bone is called its _____.

5. The muscle that contracts to produce a particular action is called the _____, or prime mover.

6. The muscle that produces the opposite movement is called the _____.

7. _____ stabilize joints so that undesirable movement does not occur.

8. _____ stabilize the origin of an agonist so that its force is fully directed onto the bone into which it inserts.

IV.   WE CAN STUDY MUSCLES IN FUNCTIONAL GROUPS

Biceps brachii	**Gluteus maximus**	**Rectus abdominis**	**Diaphragm**
Masseter	**Trapezius**	**Gastrocnemius**	**Pectoralis**

1. The _____ raises the jaw.

2. The _____ draws the shoulder upward.

3. The _____ compresses abdominal contents.

4. The _____ increases the volume of the chest cavity.

5. The _____ rotates the arm medially.

6. The _____ flexes the elbow.

7. The _____ extends and rotates the thigh.

8. The _____ flexes the foot.

Labeling Exercise

Please fill in the correct labels for Figure 5-1.

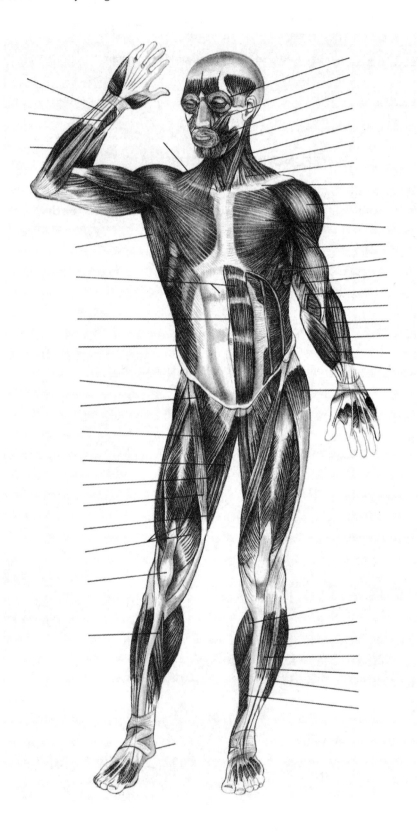

Figure 5-1

Labeling Exercise

Please fill in the correct labels for Figure 5-2.

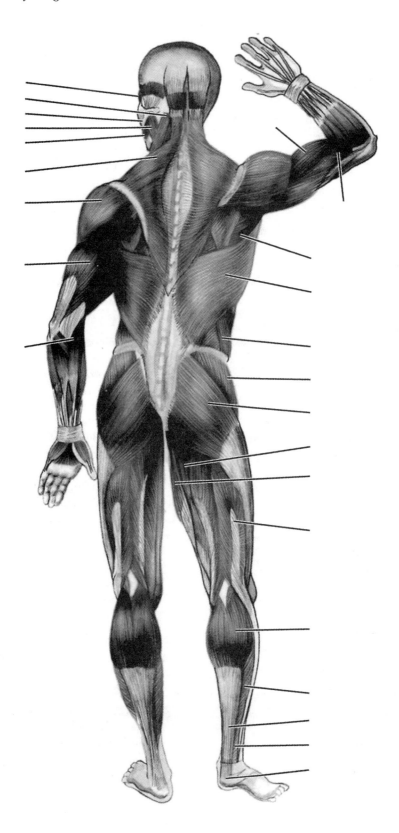

Figure 5-2

CHAPTER TEST

Select the correct response.

1. _____ depend(s) on muscle action.
   a. Walking
   b. Talking
   c. Breathing
   d. All of the above

2. Each muscle is surrounded by a covering of connective tissue called the
   a. epimysium.
   b. fascicles.
   c. perimysium.
   d. endomysium.

3. The muscle fibers are arranged in bundles called
   a. epimysium.
   b. fascicles.
   c. perimysium.
   d. endomysium.

4. Each fascicle is wrapped by connective tissue called the
   a. epimysium.
   b. myosin.
   c. perimysium.
   d. endomysium.

5. Individual muscle fibers are surrounded by a connective tissue covering called the
   a. epimysium.
   b. fascicles.
   c. perimysium.
   d. endomysium.

6. Extensions of the epimysium form tough cords of connective tissue called _____ that anchor muscles to bones.
   a. fibers
   b. tendons
   c. nerves
   d. anchors

7. Each muscle fiber is a spindle-shaped cell with many control centers called
   a. cell walls.
   b. nuclei.
   c. Golgi complexes.
   d. mitochondria.

8. Each muscle fiber is almost entirely filled with tiny protein threads, or
   a. monofilaments.
   b. striations.
   c. myofibrils.
   d. filaments.

9. Thick filaments consist mainly of the protein
   a. actin.
   b. thicktin.
   c. myosin.
   d. glycogen.

10. Thin filaments consist mainly of the protein
    a. actin.
    b. thicktin.
    c. myosin.
    d. glycogen.

11. A _____ nerve is a nerve that controls muscle contraction.
    a. controller
    b. motor
    c. contractor
    d. constrictor

12. The impulse generated during an action potential spreads through the T tubules and stimulates the release of
    a. calcium.
    b. vitamin C.
    c. acetylcholine.
    d. sodium.

13. The immediate source of energy for muscle contraction comes from the energy storage molecule,
    a. DNA.
    b. TAP.
    c. PTA.
    d. ATP.

14. Glucose is stored in muscle cells in the form of a large molecule called
    a. glycerol.
    b. glucosis.
    c. glycogen.
    d. ATP.

15. Even when we are not moving, our muscles are in a state of partial contraction called
    a. muscle tone.
    b. muscle contraction.
    c. partial tone.
    d. semicontraction.

16. When the motor nerve to a muscle is cut, the muscle becomes
    a. tight.
    b. limp.
    c. firm.
    d. stiff.

17. When a heavy object is lifted, muscles shorten and thicken as they contract. This kind of muscle contraction is called a(n) _____ contraction.
    a. isotonic
    b. isometric
    c. hypertonic
    d. hypotonic

18. When one pushes against a wall, no movement occurs, and muscle length does not appreciably change, but muscle tension increases. This type of muscle contraction is called _____ contraction.
    a. isotonic
    b. isometric
    c. hypertonic
    d. hypotonic

19. Skeletal muscles produce movements by pulling on tendons, which in turn pull on
    a. ligaments.
    b. joints.
    c. bones.
    d. other muscles.

20. The attachment of a muscle to a less movable bone is called its
    a. insertion.
    b. origin.
    c. root.
    d. inclusion.

21. The attachment of a muscle to a more movable bone is called its
    a. insertion.
    b. origin.
    c. root.
    d. inclusion.

CROSSWORD PUZZLE FOR CHAPTERS 4 AND 5

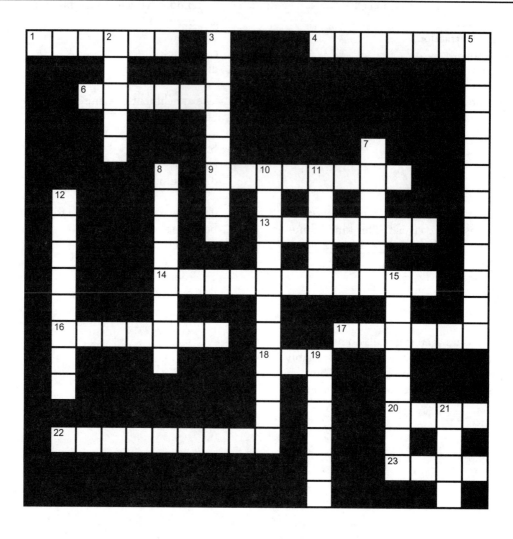

Across

1. A protein that together with actin is responsible for muscle contraction
4. Shoulder blade
6. _____ tone is the state of partial contraction that keeps muscle prepared for action
9. There are 12 _____ vertebrae
13. Three-headed muscle in posterior part of the arm
14. Cells that produce bone
16. The skull is formed by the _____ and facial bones
17. There are five _____ vertebrae
18. Immediate source of energy for muscle contraction
20. There are 12 pairs of _____
22. Each muscle fiber contains thick myosin and thin actin
23. A _____ bone consists of a shaft with flared ends

Down

2. Formed by the cranial and facial bones
3. System that supports and protects the body
5. The _____ skeleton consists of the upper and lower limbs, pectoral girdle, and pelvic girdle
7. A skeletal muscle consists of hundreds of _____ arranged in fascicles
8. In _____ contraction, muscles shorten and thicken as they contract
10. Cells that break down bone
11. The _____ skeleton consists of the skull, vertebral column, ribs, and sternum
12. There are seven _____ vertebrae
15. The cranium includes the frontal, occipital, ethmoid, spheroid, and paired parietal and _____ bones
19. The _____ girdle consists of the coxal bones together with the sacrum and coccyx
21. Compact _____ consists of osteons

Chapter

THE CENTRAL NERVOUS SYSTEM

■ ■ ■

Outline

I. The nervous system has two main divisions.
II. Neurons and glial cells are the cells of the nervous system.
III. Bundles of axons make up nerves.
IV. Appropriate responses depend on neural signaling.
V. Neurons use electrical signals to transmit information.
   A. The neuron has a resting potential.
   B. An action potential is a wave of depolarization.
VI. Neurons signal other cells across synapses.
   A. Neurons use neurotransmitters to signal other cells.
   B. Neurotransmitters bind with receptors on postsynaptic neurons.
   C. Neurotransmitter receptors can send excitatory or inhibitory signals.
VII. Neural impulses must be integrated.
VIII. The human brain is the most complex mechanism known.
   A. The medulla contains vital centers.

B. The pons is a bridge to other parts of the brain.
C. The midbrain contains centers for visual and auditory reflexes.
D. The diencephalon includes the thalamus and hypothalamus.
E. The cerebellum is responsible for coordination of movement.
F. The cerebrum is the largest part of the brain.
G. The limbic system affects emotional aspects of behavior.
H. Learning involves many areas of the brain.
IX. The spinal cord transmits information to and from the brain.
X. The central nervous system is well-protected.
   A. The meninges are connective tissue coverings.
   B. The cerebrospinal fluid cushions the CNS.
XI. A reflex action is a simple neural response.

Learning Objectives

After you have studied this chapter, you should be able to:

1. Distinguish between the central nervous system and the peripheral nervous system, and describe each.
2. Draw a neuron, label its parts, and give the functions of each.
3. Distinguish between nerve and tract; ganglion and nucleus.
4. Briefly describe the four basic processes on which all neural responses depend—reception, transmission, integration, and response.

5. Contrast the resting potential of a neuron with an action potential, and describe each.
6. Compare continuous conduction and saltatory conduction.
7. Describe the transmission of a signal across a synapse, drawing a diagram to support your description.
8. Describe the actions of the neurotransmitters discussed in this chapter.
9. Describe how a postsynaptic neuron integrates incoming stimuli and "decides" whether to fire.

10. Label on a diagram the structures of the brain described in this chapter.
11. Describe the structure and functions of the main parts of the brain: medulla, pons, midbrain, diencephalon (thalamus and hypothalamus), cerebellum, and cerebrum.
12. Name the principal areas and functions associated with the lobes of the cerebrum and the limbic system.
13. List two functions of the spinal cord and describe its structure.
14. Describe the structures that protect the brain and spinal cord.
15. Diagram a withdrawal reflex, identifying the essential structures and indicating the direction of impulse transmission.

STUDY QUESTIONS

Within each category, fill in the blanks with the correct response.

I. THE NERVOUS SYSTEM HAS TWO MAIN DIVISIONS

Afferent	**Central**	**Homeostasis**	**Somatic**	**Autonomic**	**Cranial**
Peripheral	**Spinal**	**Brain**	**Efferent**	**Sense**	

1. The two principal divisions of the nervous system are the _____ nervous system and

   the _____ nervous system.

2. The central nervous system consists of the _____ and spinal cord.

3. The peripheral nervous system is made up of the _____ organs and the nerves that are the communication lines to and from the central nervous system.

4. Twelve pairs of _____ nerves link the brain and 31 pairs of

   _____ nerves link the spinal cord with sense organs, muscles, and other parts of the body.

5. The peripheral nervous system may be subdivided into _____ and

   _____ divisions.

6. _____ (also called sensory) nerves transmit messages from sensory receptors to the central nervous system.

7. _____ (also called motor) nerves transmit information back from the central nervous system to the structures that must respond.

II. NEURONS AND GLIAL CELLS ARE THE CELLS OF THE NERVOUS SYSTEM

Axon	**Fibers**	**Myelin**	**Neurotransmitters**	**Cellular**	**Glial**
Neurilemma	**Sheath**	**Dendrites**	**Impulses**	**Neurons**	

1. _____ cells protect and support the neurons.

2. _____ are cells that are highly specialized to receive and transmit messages in the form of neural impulses.

3. The neuron is distinguished from all other cells by its _____.

4. _____ are highly branched fibers that project from the cell body and are highly specialized to receive neural impulses.

5. The single _____ transmits neural messages from the cell body toward another neuron.

6. Synaptic terminals release _____, chemical compounds that transmit impulses from one neuron to another.

7. Axons of many neurons of the peripheral nervous system are covered by two sheaths: an inner

   _____ sheath and an outer _____ sheath called a neuri-lemma.

8. The cellular _____ is important in the repair of injured neurons.

9. Myelin is an excellent electrical insulator that speeds the conduction of nerve _____.

Labeling Exercise

Please fill in the correct labels for Figure 6-1.

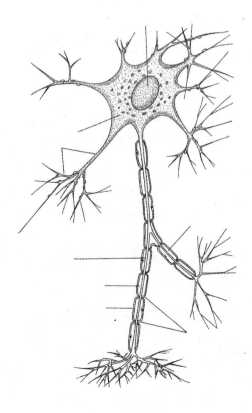

Figure 6-1

III. BUNDLES OF AXONS MAKE UP NERVES

Axons   Myelin   Nuclei   Ganglion   Nerve   Tracts

1. A(n) _____ is a large bundle of axons wrapped in connective tissue.

2. In comparing a nerve to a telephone cable, the _____ are like the individual wires,

    whereas the _____, cellular, and connective tissue sheaths are like the insulation.

3. The cell bodies attached to the axons of a nerve are often grouped together in a mass called a

    _____.

4. Within the central nervous system, bundles of axons are called _____ instead of
    nerves.

5. Within the central nervous system, masses of cell bodies are called _____ rather than
    ganglia.

IV. APPROPRIATE RESPONSES DEPEND ON NEURAL SIGNALING

1. Number the following processes in order of occurrence from 1 to 5.

    _____ Integration

    _____ Reception

    _____ Transmission (to the muscles)

    _____ Transmission (to the central nervous system)

    _____ Actual response

Dendrites   Neurotransmitters   Synaptic   Interneurons   Synapse

2. Afferent neurons transmit information to _____ in the central nervous system.

3. Neurons are arranged so that the axon of one neuron signals the _____ of other
    neurons.

4. A junction between two neurons is called a _____.

5. At a synapse, neurons are separated by a tiny gap called the _____ cleft.

6. _____ conduct "messages" across the synaptic cleft.

V.   NEURONS USE ELECTRICAL SIGNALS TO TRANSMIT INFORMATION

Plasma   Polarized   Potential

1. Most cells have a difference in electrical charge across the _____ membrane.

2. The plasma membrane is said to be electrically _____.

3. The voltage measured across the plasma membrane is referred to as the membrane

    _____.

A.   The Neuron Has a Resting Potential

Millivolts   Potassium   Sodium   Passive ion   Resting   Sodium-potassium

1. The membrane potential in a resting neuron is called its _____ potential.

2. The resting potential is generally expressed in units called _____.

3. Ions pass through specific _____ channels.

4. The gradients that determine the resting potential are maintained by _____ pumps in the plasma membrane.

5. Sodium-potassium pumps continuously transport _____ ions out of the neuron and

    _____ ions in.

B.   An Action Potential Is a Wave of Depolarization

Action potential   Permeability   Unmyelinated   Hyperpolarization
Ranvier   Voltage-activated   Impulses   Repolarization

1. Neurons have the ability to respond to stimuli and to convert stimuli into nerve

    _____.

2. An electrical, chemical, or mechanical stimulus may alter the resting potential by increasing the membrane's

    _____ to sodium.

3. _____ decreases the ability of the neuron to generate a neural impulse and is described as inhibitory.

4. When a stimulus is sufficiently strong, _____ ion channels in the plasma membrane open.

5. When voltage across the membrane is decreased to a critical point, called the threshold level, an

_____ is generated.

6. As the action potential moves down the axon, _____ occurs behind it.

7. Continuous conduction occurs in _____ neurons.

8. Myelin acts as an effective electrical insulator around the axon except at the nodes of

_____, which are not myelinated.

VI. NEURONS SIGNAL OTHER CELLS ACROSS SYNAPSES

Postsynaptic   Synapse   Presynaptic   Synaptic cleft

1. A _____ is a junction between two neurons or between a neuron and a muscle (or gland).

2. A neuron that terminates at a specific synapse is referred to as a _____ neuron.

3. A neuron that begins at a synapse is known as a _____ neuron.

4. Presynaptic and postsynaptic neurons are separated by the _____.

A.   Neurons Use Neurotransmitters to Signal Other Cells

Adrenergic	Chemical	Enkephalins	Nitric oxide	Cholinergic
Endorphins	Amino	Catecholamines	Neurotransmitters	Neuromodulators

1. _____ are chemical messengers that transmit the neural signal across the synapse to other neurons.

2. More than 60 different _____ compounds are now known to function as neurotransmitters.

3. _____ are messengers that modify the effects of specific neurotransmitters.

4. Cells that release the neurotransmitter acetylcholine are referred to as _____ neurons.

5. Neurons that release norepinephrine are called _____ neurons.

6. Norepinephrine, serotonin, and dopamine belong to a class of compounds called

_____.

7. Certain _____ acids also serve as neurotransmitters.

8. The body makes its own opioids, called _____ and _____.

9. _____ is a gas that may act as a retrograde messenger, transmitting information in the opposite direction of other neurotransmitters.

B.   Neurotransmitters Bind With Receptors on Postsynaptic Neurons

Dopamine   Receptors   Synaptic vesicles   Ion   Reuptake

1. Neurotransmitters are stored in the synaptic terminals within small membrane-bounded sacs called _____.

2. Neurotransmitter molecules diffuse across the synaptic cleft and combine with specific

    _____ on the plasma membranes of postsynaptic cells.

3. Neurotransmitter receptors are chemically activated _____ channels.

4. _____ is the process where catecholamines are actively transported back into the synaptic terminals.

5. Cocaine inhibits the reuptake of _____.

C.   Neurotransmitter Receptors Can Send Excitatory or Inhibitory Signals

Summation   Inhibitory postsynaptic potential (IPSP)   Excitatory
Inhibitory   Excitatory postsynaptic potential (EPSP)

1. Acetylcholine has a(n) _____ effect on skeletal muscle, while it has a(n)

    _____ effect on cardiac muscle.

2. A change in membrane potential that brings the neuron closer to firing is called a(n)

    _____.

3. A(n) _____ occurs when a neurotransmitter-receptor combination hyperpolarizes the postsynaptic membrane, taking the neuron farther away from the firing level.

4. Excitatory postsynaptic potentials may be added together in a process known as

    _____.

VII. NEURAL IMPULSES MUST BE INTEGRATED

Neural integration Cancel Graded Action potential CNS

1. _____ is the process of summing incoming signals.

2. EPSPs and IPSPs are produced continually in postsynaptic neurons, and IPSPs _____ the effects of some of the EPSPs.

3. IPSPs and EPSPs are _____ responses that may be added to or subtracted from other EPSPs and IPSPs.

4. Local responses permit the neuron and the entire nervous system a far greater range of response than would

    be the case if every EPSP generated a(n) _____.

5. Most neural integration takes place in the _____.

VIII. THE HUMAN BRAIN IS THE MOST COMPLEX MECHANISM KNOWN

Cerebrovascular Neural Stroke Glucose Oxygen Ventricles

1. At any given moment, millions of _____ messages are flashing through the brain.

2. Brain cells require a continuous supply of _____ and _____.

3. The most common cause of brain damage is a _____.

4. In a(n) _____ accident, a portion of the brain is deprived of its blood supply.

5. The brain is a hollow organ; its fluid-filled spaces are called _____.

A. The Medulla Contains Vital Centers

Cardiac   Oblongata   Spinal cord   Cerebrum   Respiratory
Vasomotor   Medulla   Reticular formation

1. Formally known as the medulla _____, the medulla is the most posterior portion of the brain stem.

2. Because of its position, all nerve tracts carrying messages from the _____ to the brain must pass through the medulla.

3. The _____ is a network of neurons that extends from the spinal cord through the medulla and upward through the brain stem and thalamus.

4. The reticular formation is important in keeping the _____ conscious and alert.

5. _____ centers in the medulla control heart rate.

6. _____ centers in the medulla regulate blood pressure by controlling the diameter of the blood vessels.

7. _____ centers in the medulla initiate and regulate breathing.

8. Four cranial nerves, designated cranial nerves IX through XII, originate within the

_____.

B.   The Pons Is a Bridge to Other Parts of the Brain

Brain   Medulla   Respiration   Cerebellum   Nerve

1. The _____ forms a bulge on the anterior (ventral) surface of the brain stem.

2. The pons is just superior to the _____, with which it is continuous.

3. The posterior surface of the pons is hidden by the _____.

4. The pons serves as a link connecting various parts of the _____.

5. The pons consists mainly of _____ fibers passing between the medulla and other parts of the brain.

6. The pons contains centers that help regulate _____ and sleep.

C.   The Midbrain Contains Centers for Visual and Auditory Reflexes

Auditory   Midbrain   Pons   Cerebral aqueduct   Neurons   Visual

1. The _____ is the shortest portion of the brain stem.

2. The midbrain extends from the _____ to the diencephalon.

3. The cavity of the midbrain is known as the _____ and connects the third and fourth ventricles.

4. The midbrain consists of large bundles of _____.

5. Reflex centers controlling _____ and _____ reflexes are located in the roof of the midbrain.

D. The Diencephalon Includes the Thalamus and the Hypothalamus

Autonomic	Endocrine	Motor	Circadian	Hypothalamus
Thalamus	Diencephalon	Motivational	Nuclei	Suprachiasmatic

1. The _____ is the part of the brain between the cerebrum and the midbrain.

2. The _____ is a major relay center, consisting of two oval masses, located on each side of the third ventricle.

3. _____ in the thalamus serve as relay stations for all sensory information (except smell) to the cerebrum.

4. The thalamus integrates motor information from the cerebellum and transmits messages to

   _____ areas in the cerebrum.

5. The _____ lies below the thalamus. Its function is to help regulate homeostasis and reproductive behavior.

6. The hypothalamus is sometimes called the control center of the _____ nervous system because it is the most important relay station between the cerebral cortex and the lower autonomic centers.

7. The hypothalamus is the link between the nervous and _____ systems.

8. The hypothalamus helps determine emotional and _____ states.

9. Along with the brain stem, the hypothalamus regulates sleep-wake cycles called

   _____ rhythms.

10. The _____ nucleus in the hypothalamus is the most important of the body's biological clocks.

E. The Cerebellum Is Responsible for Coordination of Movement

Cerebellum   Motor   Muscle   Language   Movements   Vestibular

1. The _____ is the second-largest part of the brain, and consists of two lateral masses called hemispheres and a connecting portion.

2. The cerebellum helps make _____ smooth instead of jerky, and steady rather than trembling.

3. The cerebellum helps maintain _____ tone and posture.

4. Impulses from the _____ apparatus in the inner ear are continuously delivered to the cerebellum, which uses that information to help maintain equilibrium.

5. The cerebellum is also important in learning _____ skills.

6. The cerebellum is also important in cognitive function, including _____.

F.   The Cerebrum Is the Largest Part of the Brain

Association   Frontal   Movement   Intellectual   Cerebrum   Corpus callosum
Temporal   Sensory   Parietal   Motor   Transverse   Primary visual area

1. The _____ is the largest and most prominent part of the human brain.

2. The functions of the cerebrum can be divided into _____ functions,

   _____ functions, and _____ functions.

3. The motor areas of the cerebrum are responsible for all voluntary and some involuntary

   _____.

4. *Association* is a term used to describe all of the _____ activities of the cerebral cortex.

5. The cerebrum is separated from the cerebellum by the _____ fissure.

6. The _____ connects the right and left hemispheres of the cerebrum.

7. The precentral gyrus is located in the _____ lobe.

8. The postcentral gyrus is located in the _____ lobe.

9. The area in the occipital lobe that receives visual information is known as the _____.

10. The _____ lobe is concerned with reception and integration of auditory messages.

G.   The Limbic System Affects Emotional Aspects of Behavior

Amygdala   Hippocampus   Memories   Emotional   Limbic   Motivation

1. The _____ system is a group of interconnected nuclei involved in memory and in
   the regulation of emotion.

2. The limbic system is responsible for evaluating awards, and is important in _____.

3. Two important limbic regions are the _____ and the _____.

4. The hippocampus is involved in the formation and retrieval of _____.

5. The amygdala is important in determining the _____ aspects of memory.

Labeling Exercise

Please fill in the correct labels for Figure 6-2.

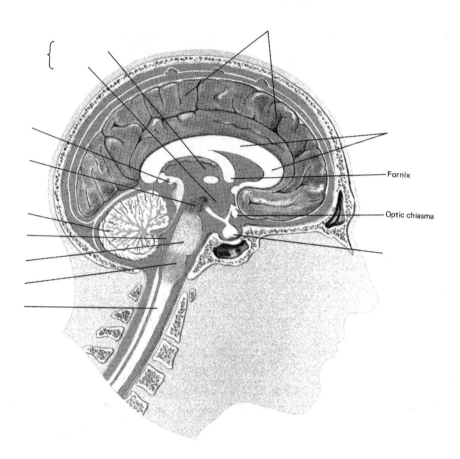

Fornix

Optic chiasma

Figure 6-2

H. Learning Involves Many Areas of the Brain

Learning   Memory   Synaptic plasticity

1. _____ is the process by which we acquire information as a result of experience.

2. _____ is the process by which information is encoded, stored, and retrieved.

3. _____ refers to the ability of the nervous system to modify synapses during learning and remembering.

IX. THE SPINAL CORD TRANSMITS INFORMATION TO AND FROM THE BRAIN

Ascending   Fissures   Vertebral   Descending   Spinal

1. The _____ cord has two main functions: (1) it controls many reflex activities of the body, and (2) it transmits information between the nerves and the peripheral nervous system of the brain.

2. The spinal cord occupies the _____ canal of the vertebral column.

3. Several grooves called _____ divide the spinal cord into regions.

4. _____ tracts transmit sensory information up the spinal cord to the brain.

5. _____ tracts transmit impulses from the brain down the spinal cord to the efferent nerves.

Labeling Exercise

Please fill in the correct labels for Figure 6-3.

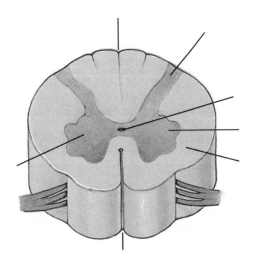

Figure 6-3

X.   THE CENTRAL NERVOUS SYSTEM IS WELL-PROTECTED

A.   The Meninges Are Connective Tissue Coverings

Arachnoid   Encephalitis   Meningitis   Sinuses   Dura mater   Meninges   Pia mater

1. The three connective tissue layers covering the brain and spinal cord are the _____.

2. The outermost layer of the meninges is the _____, a tough, double-layered membrane.

3. Inside the skull, the two layers of the dura mater are separated in some regions by large blood vessels called

    _____. These vessels receive blood leaving the brain and deliver it to the jugular veins in the neck.

4. The second layer of the meninges is the _____, a thin, delicate membrane.

5. The innermost meningeal layer is the _____, a very thin membrane that adheres closely to the brain and spinal cord.

6. _____ is an inflammation of the meninges.

7. Some viruses that cause meningitis can spread, causing inflammation of the brain itself. This more serious illness is _____.

B. The Cerebrospinal Fluid Cushions the CNS

Brain   Choroid plexuses   Lumbar   Cerebrospinal fluid   Hydrocephalus

1. The shock-absorbing fluid that fills the ventricles (the cavities within the brain) and the spaces below the arachnoid layer in the brain and spinal cord is called _____.

2. Most of the cerebrospinal fluid (CSF) is produced by clusters of capillaries called the _____.

3. The _____ actually floats in CSF, which protects it against mechanical injury.

4. Abnormally rapid production of CSF can result in _____.

5. A _____ puncture is a procedure that can be used to withdraw small amounts of CSF or measure CSF pressure without damaging the spinal cord.

XI. A REFLEX ACTION IS A SIMPLE NEURAL RESPONSE

Inhibit   Reflex   Regulation

1. A simple example of a neural response is a(n) _____ action.

2. A good example of a reflex action is the _____ of body temperature.

3. We can consciously _____ or facilitate some reflexes.

Labeling Exercise

Please fill in the correct labels for Figure 6-4.

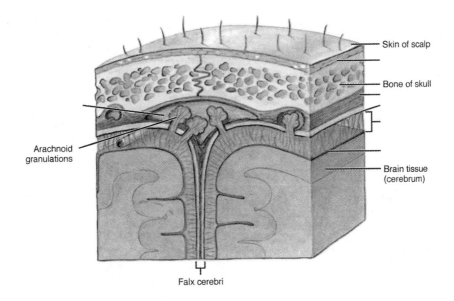

Skin of scalp

Bone of skull

Brain tissue
(cerebrum)

Arachnoid
granulations

Falx cerebri

Figure 6-4

CHAPTER TEST

Select the correct response.

1. The _____ system serves as the body's link to
    the outside world.
    a. digestive
    b. nervous
    c. reproductive
    d. circulatory

2. The two principal divisions of the nervous
    system are the
    a. central and accessory nervous systems.
    b. central and autonomic nervous systems.
    c. central and peripheral nervous systems.
    d. autonomic and peripheral nervous systems.

3. The central nervous system is made up of the
    a. eyes and ears.
    b. brain and spinal cord.
    c. taste buds.
    d. both a and c.

4. The peripheral nervous system includes the
    a. sense organs (i.e., eyes, ears, etc.).
    b. arms and legs.
    c. heart and lungs.
    d. muscles and bones.

5. The correct order of response of the following
    processes is
    a. reception, transmission, integration, trans-
        mission, response.
    b. transmission, reception, transmission,
        integration, response.
    c. reception, integration, transmission, re-
        sponse, transmission.
    d. response, reception, transmission, integra-
        tion, transmission.

6. The main divisions of the brain are the
    a. medulla, pons, diencephalon, and cerebrum.
    b. medulla, pons, midbrain, diencephalon,
        cerebrum, and cerebellum.
    c. medulla, cerebrum, and cerebellum.
    d. thalamus, hypothalamus, medulla, and
        cerebrum.

7. The brain stem is made up of the
    a. medulla, pons, and cerebrum.
    b. cerebellum, midbrain, and pons.
    c. medulla, pons, and midbrain.
    d. midbrain, pons, and cerebrum.

8. The _____ is a vital center of the medulla.
   a. cardiac center
   b. vasomotor center
   c. respiratory center
   d. all of the above

9. All of the following are functions of the hypothalamus except
   a. linking nervous and endocrine systems.
   b. helping to maintain fluid balance.
   c. regulating body temperature.
   d. coordination of movement.

10. Functions of the cerebellum include helping to
    a. smooth and coordinate movement.
    b. maintain posture.
    c. maintain equilibrium.
    d. all of the above.

11. All of the following are functions of the cerebrum except
    a. controlling motor activities.
    b. interpreting sensation.
    c. serving as the center of intellect.
    d. regulating body temperature.

12. Which of the following processes are components of a reflex pathway?
    a. reception of the stimulus
    b. transmission of information
    c. integration of the stimulus
    d. all of the above

Chapter

THE PERIPHERAL NERVOUS SYSTEM

■ ■ ■

Outline

Introduction

I. The somatic division responds to changes in the outside world.
  A. Cranial nerves link the brain with sensory receptors and muscles.
  B. Spinal nerves link the spinal cord with various structures.
    1. Each spinal nerve divides into branches and the ventral branches form plexuses.

II. The autonomic division maintains internal balance.
  A. The sympathetic system mobilizes energy.
  B. The parasympathetic system conserves and restores energy.

Learning Objectives

After you have studied this chapter, you should be able to:

1. Contrast the somatic with the autonomic divisions of the peripheral nervous system.
2. List the cranial nerves and give the functions of each.
3. Describe the structure of a typical spinal nerve.
4. Name and describe the major plexuses.
5. Describe a reflex pathway in the autonomic system.

6. Compare and contrast the sympathetic system with the parasympathetic system.
7. Compare the effect of sympathetic stimulation with that of parasympathetic stimulation on specific organs such as the heart and the digestive tract.

STUDY QUESTIONS

Within each category, fill in the blanks with the correct response.

INTRODUCTION

Autonomic   Sensory   Somatic

1. The peripheral nervous system is made up of _____ receptors, the nerves that link the sense organs with the central nervous system, and the nerves that link the central nervous system with the muscles and glands.

2. The portion of the peripheral nervous system that keeps the body in adjustment with the outside world is

   the _____ system.

3. The nerves and receptors that maintain internal balance make up the _____ system.

I. THE SOMATIC DIVISION RESPONDS TO CHANGES IN THE OUTSIDE WORLD

Cranial   Spinal   Somatic

1. The _____ division includes the sensory receptors that react to changes in the outside world.

2. The afferent and efferent neurons of the somatic system, like those of the autonomic division, are part of the

   _____ and _____ nerves.

A.   Cranial Nerves Link the Brain With Sensory Receptors and Muscles

Afferent   Cranial   Sensory   CNS   Efferent

1. Twelve pairs of _____ nerves emerge form the brain.

2. Cranial nerves transmit information to the brain from _____ receptors.

3. Cranial nerves transmit orders from the _____ to muscles and glands.

4. Most cranial nerves consist of both sensory (or _____) neurons, and motor (or

   _____) neurons.

B.   Spinal Nerves Link the Spinal Cord With Various Structures

Coccygeal   Five   Spinal   Vertebral column   Dorsal
Ganglion   Thoracic   Eight   Lumbar   Ventral

1. Thirty-one pairs of _____ nerves emerge form the spinal cord.

2. Spinal nerves are named for the general region of the _____ from which they originate and are numbered in sequence.

3. There are _____ pairs of cervical spinal nerves.

4. There are 12 pairs of _____ spinal nerves.

5. There are five pairs of _____ spinal nerves.

6. There are _____ pairs of sacral spinal nerves.

7. There is one pair of _____ spinal nerves.

8. The _____ root consists of afferent fibers that transmit information from sensory receptors to the spinal cord.

9. Just before the dorsal root joins the spinal cord, it is marked by a swelling called the spinal

    _____, which consists of the cell bodies of the sensory neurons.

10. The _____ root consists of efferent fibers leaving the spinal cord.

1. Each Spinal Nerve Divides Into Branches and the Ventral Branches Form Plexuses

Brachial   Dorsal   Lumbar   Sciatic   Branches   Femoral   Plexuses   Ventral   Cervical   Innervate   Sacral

1. Just after a spinal nerve emerges form the vertebral column, it divides into _____.

2. The _____ branch of each nerve supplies the muscles and skin of the posterior part of the body in that region.

3. The _____ branch innervates the anterior and lateral body trunk in that area as well as the limbs.

4. The ventral branches of several spinal nerves interconnect forming networks called

    _____.

5. Nerves that emerge from a plexus may be named for the region of the body that they

    _____.

6. The main plexuses are the _____ plexus, the _____ plexus,

    the _____ plexus, and the _____ plexus.

7. The _____ nerve is the largest nerve arising from the lumbar plexus.

8. The main branch of the sacral plexus is the _____ nerve, the largest nerve in the body.

Labeling Exercise

Please fill in the correct labels for Figure 7-1.

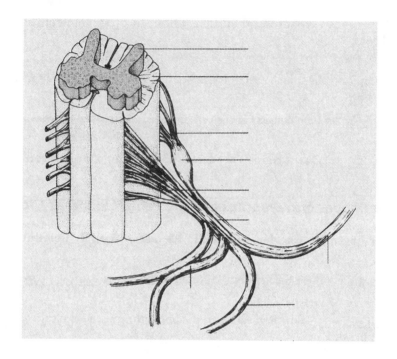

Figure 7-1

II. THE AUTONOMIC DIVISION MAINTAINS INTERNAL BALANCE

Autonomic   Efferent   Parasympathetic   Sympathetic

1. The _____ division works automatically to maintain a steady state within the body.

2. The efferent portion of the autonomic division is subdivided into _____ and

   _____ systems.

3. In the autonomic division, two _____ neurons are found between the central nervous system and the muscle it innervates.

A. The Sympathetic System Mobilizes Energy

Acetylcholine   Cholinergic   Norepinephrine   Preganglionic   Action   Collateral
Paravertebral   Sympathetic   Adrenergic   Neurons   Postganglionic

1. The sympathetic system prepares the body for _____.

2. The _____ system dominates when you are rushing to class or taking a test.

3. _____ of the sympathetic system emerge from the thoracic and lumbar regions of the spinal cord.

4. Efferent sympathetic neurons pass through the autonomic branch of the spinal nerve, then they pass into the ganglia of the _____ sympathetic ganglion chain.

5. Some of the first efferent neurons pass on to ganglia located in the abdomen, known as _____ ganglia.

6. The first efferent neurons are referred to as _____ neurons.

7. The second efferent neurons are referred to as _____ neurons.

8. Preganglionic neurons of the sympathetic system release the neurotransmitter _____, and are referred to as _____.

9. Postganglionic neurons release _____, and are referred to as _____.

B.   The Parasympathetic System Conserves and Restores Energy

Acetylcholine   Conserving   Terminal ganglia   Active   Parasympathetic   Vagus   Brain   Pelvic

1. The parasympathetic system is most _____ during periods of calm and physical rest.

2. Activities of the parasympathetic system result in _____ and restoring energy.

3. Neurons of the parasympathetic system emerge from the _____ and from the sacral region of the spinal cord.

4. Most of the parasympathetic fibers are in the _____ nerves.

5. The first efferent neurons synapse with the second efferent neurons in _____ located near or within the walls of the organs they innervate.

6. The parasympathetic nerves that emerge from the sacral region form the _____ nerves.

7. _____ nerves do not innervate blood vessels or sweat glands.

8. Both preganglionic and postganglionic fibers of the parasympathetic system release the neurotransmitter _____. They are cholinergic.

CHAPTER TEST

Select the correct response.

1. The _____ nerves link the brain with sense receptors and muscles.
   a. cranial
   b. spinal
   c. thalamic
   d. thoracic

2. There are 8 pairs of _____ spinal nerves and 12 pairs _____ of spinal nerves.
   a. cervical; sacral
   b. lumbar; thoracic
   c. cervical; thoracic
   d. thoracic; lumbar

3. The _____ ganglion consists of cell bodies of sensory neurons.
   a. paravertebral
   b. spinal
   c. ventral
   d. collateral

4. The ventral branches of several spinal nerves interconnect, forming networks called
   a. ganglia.
   b. tracts.
   c. cranial nerves.
   d. plexuses.

5. The _____ plexus supplies the thigh, leg, and foot.
   a. brachial
   b. cervical
   c. lumbar
   d. sacral

6. The main branch of the sacral plexus is the _____ nerve.
   a. cardiac
   b. vagus
   c. sciatic
   d. phrenic

7. In the autonomic division, two _____ neurons are found between the central nervous system and the muscle it innervates.
   a. afferent
   b. efferent
   c. sensory
   d. cranial

8. _____ nerves increase heart rate.
   a. Sympathetic
   b. Parasympathetic
   c. Vagus
   d. Spinal

9. In the sympathetic system, some efferent neurons end in _____ ganglia located in the abdomen.
   a. collateral
   b. terminal
   c. paravertebral
   d. spinal

10. Neurons of the sympathetic system emerge from the _____ and _____ regions of the spinal cord.
    a. cervical; thoracic
    b. thoracic; lumbar
    c. lumbar; sacral
    d. cervical; lumbar

11. The _____ system is most active during periods of calm.
    a. somatic
    b. parasympathetic
    c. sympathetic
    d. cranial

12. In the parasympathetic system, the first efferent neurons synapse with the second efferent neurons in _____ ganglia.
    a. collateral
    b. terminal
    c. paravertebral
    d. spinal

Chapter

THE SENSE ORGANS

■ ■ ■

Outline

Introduction
I. Sensory receptors produce receptor potentials.
II. We can classify sensory receptors according to the type of energy they transduce.
III. The eye contains photoreceptors.
   A. The eye can be compared to a camera.
   B. The retina contains light-sensitive rods and cones.
   C. The optic nerve transmits signals to the brain.
IV. The ear functions in hearing and equilibrium.
   A. The outer ear conducts sound waves to the middle ear.
   B. The middle ear amplifies sound waves.
   C. The inner ear contains mechanoreceptors.
     1. The cochlea contains the receptors for hearing.

     2. Sounds vary in pitch, loudness, and quality.
     3. The vestibule and semicircular canals help maintain equilibrium.
V. Smell is sensed by chemoreceptors in the nasal cavity.
VI. Taste buds detect dissolved food molecules.
VII. The general senses are widespread throughout the body.
   A. Tactile receptors are located in the skin.
   B. Temperature receptors are nerve endings.
   C. Pain sensation is a protective mechanism.
   D. Proprioceptors inform us of our position.

Learning Objectives

After you have studied this chapter, you should be able to:

1. Describe how a sensory receptor functions.
2. Compare four types of sensory receptors classified according to the type of energy they transduce.
3. Describe the structures of the eye and give their functions. (Include a description of the neural pathway.)
4. Describe the structures and functions of the three major parts of the ear.
5. Trace the transmission of sound through the ear.

6. Describe the functions of the vestibule and semicircular canals.
7. Compare the receptors of taste and smell.
8. Describe the tactile receptors and temperature receptors.
9. Describe the process of pain perception and explain the basis of phantom and referred pain.
10. Locate proprioceptors in the body and describe their functions.

STUDY QUESTIONS

Within each category, fill in the blanks with the correct response.

INTRODUCTION

Ears   Receptors   Taste buds   Eyes   Sensory   Nose   Stimulus

1. Any detectable change in the environment is called a _____.

2. We detect stimuli through our _____ receptors.

3. Sensory receptors, along with other types of cells, make up complex sense organs such as

    _____, _____, _____, and

    _____.

4. How we respond to changes in our environment depends on _____ that sense changes in the outside world as well as inside our bodies.

I.   SENSORY RECEPTORS PRODUCE RECEPTOR POTENTIALS

CNS   Receptor potential   Transduction   Depolarized   Stimulus

1. Sensory receptors absorb a small amount of energy from some _____ in the environment.

2. In a process known as _____, sensory receptors convert the energy of a stimulus into electrical energy.

3. Sensory receptors produce a _____, a depolarization or hyperpolarization of the membrane.

4. When a sensory receptor is _____, an action potential may be initiated in a sensory neuron.

5. Sensory neurons transmit information from the receptors to the _____.

II.   WE CAN CLASSIFY SENSORY RECEPTORS ACCORDING TO THE TYPE OF ENERGY THEY TRANSDUCE

Chemoreceptors   Photoreceptors   Mechanoreceptors   Thermoreceptors

1. _____ transduce mechanical energy such as touch, pressure, or gravity.

2. _____ transduce chemical compounds.

3. _____ transduce light energy.

4. _____ respond to heat and cold.

III.   THE EYE CONTAINS PHOTORECEPTORS

Extrinsic	Pupil	Blinking	Conjunctiva	Lacrimal glands	Iris
Eyelashes	Reflex	Choroid	Eyelids	Vitreous humor	Sclera
Retina	Light	Fat	Lacrimal ducts	Suspensory ligament	
Orbit	Cornea	Lens	Aqueous humor		

1. The eye and its muscles are set in the _____ formed by the skeletal bones of the face.

2. The eye and its muscles are cushioned by layers of _____.

3. The _____ and _____ help protect the eye anteriorly from foreign objects.

4. The eyelids close by _____ action if danger is perceived.

5. Frequent _____ of the eye lubricates the eye and clears debris.

6. Tears flow at all times from the _____.

7. Tears pass through the _____ to keep the eye moist and free from dust and minute objects.

8. The six _____ muscles of the eye originate from outside the eye and function in support and movement.

9. The eyeball is formed by three layers of tissue: the fibrous sclera and _____, the _____ layer, and the _____.

10. The _____ is known as the "white of the eye."

11. The sclera is covered by the _____, a moist mucous membrane that extends as a continuous lining of the inner layer of the eyelids.

12. The _____ is the colored part of the eye.

13. The iris regulates the amount of _____ entering the eye.

14. The black spot in the middle of the eye is called the _____.

15. The _____ of the eye is a transparent, elastic ball that lies at the rear of the anterior cavity of the eyeball.

16. The anterior cavity between the cornea and the lens is filled with a watery substance known as the

   _____.

17. The larger posterior cavity between the lens and the retina is filled with a more viscous fluid known as the

   _____.

18. The lens is attached to the ciliary muscles by tiny fibers that make up the _____.

A. The Eye Can Be Compared to a Camera

Accommodation   Ovoid   Relaxes   Ciliary   Presbyopia   Retina

1. The _____ can be compared to the light-sensitive film used in a camera.

2. The ability of the eye to change focus for near or far vision by changing the shape of the lens is called

   _____.

3. To focus on objects that are near, the _____ muscle contracts.

4. To focus on distant objects, the ciliary muscle _____ and the lens assumes a

   flattened, or _____, shape.

5. _____ occurs with age and results in the loss of elasticity of the lens, causing it to fail
   to focus properly on an object.

B. The Retina Contains Light-Sensitive Rods and Cones

Bipolar   Ganglion   Photoreceptors   Cones   Optic   Rhodopsin   Fovea   Optic disc   Rods

1. The retina contains _____ called rods and cones.

2. The _____ are responsible for color vision and vision during daytime.

3. The _____ are responsible for vision in dim light or darkness.

4. Cones are most concentrated in the _____, a small depression in the center of the
   posterior region of the retina.

5. Photoreceptors synapse on _____ cells, which make synaptic contact with

   _____ cells.

6. The axons of the ganglion cells extend across the surface of the retina and unite to form the

   _____ nerve.

7. The area where the optic nerve passes out of the eyeball, the _____, is known as the blind spot because it lacks rods and cones.

8. The breakdown of the pigment _____ leads to the transduction of light and the transmission of neural signals.

C.   The Optic Nerve Transmits Signals to the Brain

Cerebrum   **Optic chiasm**   **Primary visual cortex**
Lateral geniculate   **Optic nerves**   **Trigeminal nerve**

1. Axons of ganglion cells in the retina form the _____ which transmit information to the brain by way of complex, encoded signals.

2. The optic nerves cross in the floor of the hypothalamus, forming an X-shaped structure called the

   _____.

3. Axons of the optic nerves end in the _____ nuclei of the thalamus.

4. From the thalamus, neurons send signals to the _____ in the occipital lobe of the cerebrum.

5. Information about touch, pain, and temperature is transmitted from the eye to the brain by the

   _____.

6. We know that a large part of the association areas of the _____ are involved in integrating visual input.

Labeling Exercise

Please fill in the correct labels for Figure 8-1.

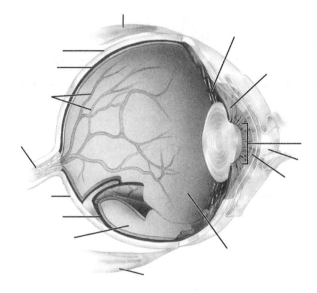

Figure 8-1

IV.   THE EAR FUNCTIONS IN HEARING AND EQUILIBRIUM

Equilibrium   Middle   Outer   Sensory

1.   The _____ ear includes the part we see and a canal connecting with the middle ear.

2.   The _____ ear contains three small bones that conduct sound waves.

3.   The inner ear contains _____ receptors for sounds waves and for maintaining the

_____ of the body.

A.   The Outer Ear Conducts Sound Waves to the Middle Ear

Cerumen   External auditory meatus   Tympanic membrane   Ceruminous   Pinna

1.   The _____ is the part of the outer ear that projects from the side of the head and
surrounds the ear canal.

2.   The ear canal, also known as the _____, leads to the middle ear.

3.   The lining of the ear canal contains _____ glands that secrete earwax.

4.   _____, commonly called earwax, helps protect the lining of the ear canal from
infection.

5.   The _____, or eardrum, separates the middle and external ear.

B.   The Middle Ear Amplifies Sound Waves

Eustachian	Middle ear	Stapes	Incus	Tympanic membrane
Ossicles	Malleus	Oval window	Vibrations	

1.   The _____ is a small, moist cavity in the temporal bone containing air and three

small bones called _____ .

2.   Under normal circumstances, air pressure is equalized on both sides of the tympanic membrane by the

_____ tube.

3.   The three auditory ossicles are the _____ , _____ , and

_____ .

4.   The auditory ossicles form a chain from the tympanic membrane to the _____ , a
small membrane between the middle and inner ear.

5.   Sound waves cause vibrations of the _____ .

6.   The auditory ossicles act as three interconnected levers that help amplify the _____ .

C.   The Inner Ear Contains Mechanoreceptors

Cochlea	Labyrinth	Vibrations	Endolymph	Mechanoreceptors
Perilymph	Equilibrium	Membranous	Vestibule	Semicircular canals

1.   The inner ear contains _____ that convert sound waves to nerve impulses.

2.   The inner ear also contains receptors that allow us to maintain our _____ .

3.   The inner ear is a bony _____ composed of three compartments.

4.   The _____ , _____ , and _____ make
up the three compartments of the inner ear.

5.   The bony labyrinth contains a fluid called _____ .

6.   The perilymph surrounds the _____ labyrinth.

7.   The membranous labyrinth contains a fluid called _____ .

8.   Perilymph and endolymph carry _____ through the system of canals within the
inner ear.

1. The Cochlea Contains the Receptors for Hearing

| Basilar | Perilymph | Vestibular | Cochlea | Hair | Cochlear nerve |
| Stereocilia | Cochlear | Tympanic | Organ of Corti | | |

1. The _____ is a snail-shaped portion of the middle ear.

2. The cochlea contains the _____, the sound receptor.

3. Sensory receptors inside the organ of Corti respond to sound waves by stimulating the

   _____.

4. The _____ canal and the _____ canal are connected at the

   apex of the cochlea and are filled with _____.

5. The _____ duct is filled with endolymph and contains the organ of Corti.

6. Each organ of Corti contains about 18,000 _____ cells arranged in rows that extend the length of the coiled cochlea.

7. Each hair cell in the organ of Corti is equipped with tiny projections called _____ that extend into the cochlear duct.

8. The _____ membrane separates the cochlear duct from the tympanic canal.

2. Sounds Vary in Pitch, Loudness, and Quality

Amplitude Hair Low-frequency Cochlear High-frequency Pitch Deafness High-intensity

1. _____ depends on frequency of sound waves and is expressed as hertz (Hz).

2. _____ vibrations result in the sensation of low pitch.

3. _____ vibrations result in the sensation of high pitch.

4. The brain infers the pitch of a sound from the particular _____ cells that are stimulated.

5. Loud sounds cause resonance waves of greater _____.

6. When the hair cells are more intensely stimulated, the _____ nerve transmits a greater number of impulses per second.

7. _____ may be caused by injury to, or malformation of, the sound-perceiving mechanism of the inner ear.

8. Exposure to _____ sound, such as heavily amplified music, damages the hair cells of the organ of Corti.

D.   The Vestibule and Semicircular Canals Help Maintain Equilibrium

Endolymph **Semicircular** **Vestibule** **Cupula** **Crista** **Angular acceleration**
Otoliths **Vestibulocochlear** **Utricle** **Saccule** **Vestibular**

1. The _____ and _____ canals contain receptor cells that transmit information about the position of the body.

2. Inside the vestibule, the membranous labyrinth is divided into two saclike chambers—the

_____ and the _____.

3. _____ are small, calcium carbonate ear stones that act as gravity detectors.

4. Each receptor cell has a group of hair cells surrounded at their tips by a gelatinous mass called a

_____.

5. Information about turning movements, referred to as _____, is provided by the three semicircular canals.

6. Within each ampulla lies a clump of hair cells called a _____.

7. The response of the sensory cells in the semicircular canals is produced by the flow of

_____ within the canals as the position of the head changes.

8. The _____ nerve joins the cochlear nerve to form the _____ nerve.

Labeling Exercise

Please fill in the correct labels for Figure 8-2.

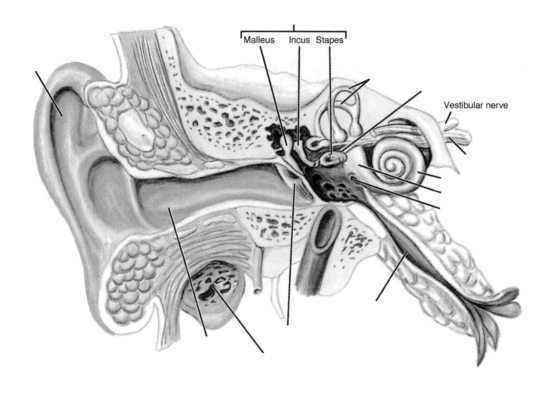

Figure 8-2

V. SMELL IS SENSED BY CHEMORECEPTORS IN THE NASAL CAVITY

Odors   Olfactory nerve   Temporal   Olfactory   Scents

1. Smell is sensed by chemoreceptor cells in the _____ epithelium at the upper part of the nasal cavity.

2. Odors detected by the olfactory epithelium are transmitted by the _____ to the

   olfactory cortex in the _____ lobe.

3. We can detect at least seven main groups of _____, and we can perceive about 10,000

   different _____.

VI.   TASTE BUDS DETECT DISSOLVED FOOD MOLECULES

Bitter	Regenerated	Sour	Gustation	Salty	Tip	Taste receptors
Sweet	Papillae	Sides	Taste	Posterior	Smell	Taste buds

1. The sense of taste, called _____, is the job of the _____ on the tongue and various parts of the mouth.

2. Taste buds are found mainly in tiny elevations, or _____, on the tongue.

3. _____ detect chemical substances dissolved in saliva.

4. Unlike most neurons, both taste and smell receptors are continuously _____.

5. Traditionally, four main tastes have been recognized: _____,

_____, _____, and _____.

6. Sweet and salty tastes are sensed mainly at the _____ of the tongue.

7. Sour taste is detected mainly at the _____ of the tongue and bitter taste is detected at

the _____ part of the tongue.

8. Both _____ and _____ are important in stimulating appetite and digestive juices.

VII.   THE GENERAL SENSES ARE WIDESPREAD THROUGHOUT THE BODY

Muscle   Pressure   Touch   Pain   Temperature   Vibration

1. The general senses include the receptors that respond to _____,

_____, _____, _____, changes in

_____, and _____ stretch.

A.   Tactile Receptors Are Located in the Skin

Mechanoreceptors   Pressure   Touch   Pain   Tactile

1. The simplest _____ are free nerve endings in the skin.

2. Free nerve endings in the skin detect _____, _____, and

_____ when stimulated by objects that contact the body surface.

3. Some of the more specialized _____ receptors located in the skin can detect light touch and pressure, whereas others inform us of heavy and continuous touch and pressure.

B. Temperature Receptors Are Nerve Endings

Homeostatic   Mouth   Thermoreceptors   Hypothalamus   Skin   Lips   Temperature

1. _____ are free nerve endings that allow us to recognize cold, cool, warm, and hot.

2. Widely distributed throughout the body, thermoreceptors are especially concentrated in the

   _____ and _____.

3. Thermoreceptors are highly sensitive to differences between _____ temperature and

   the _____ of objects that come into contact with the body.

4. Thermoreceptors in the _____ detect internal changes in temperature and receive and integrate information from thermoreceptors on the body surface. The hypothalamus then initiates

   _____ mechanisms that ensure a constant body temperature.

C. Pain Sensation Is a Protective Mechanism

Acupuncture   Enkephalins   Nociceptors   Referred   Analgesia   Glutamate
Substance P   Mechanical   Phantom pain   Pain   Thermal   Beta-endorphins

1. The sensation of _____ is a protective mechanism that makes us aware of tissue injury.

2. Pain receptors, called _____, are free nerve endings of certain sensory neurons found in almost every tissue.

3. _____ nociceptors respond to temperature extremes.

4. _____ nociceptors respond to strong tactile stimuli such as penetration by sharp objects or pinching.

5. The sensory neurons release the neurotransmitter _____ and several other

   neurotransmitters, including _____.

6. The body has a variety of mechanisms for _____, or pain control.

7. _____ and _____ are among the more than 10 opiates that exist in the brain, spinal cord, and pituitary gland.

8. For years after an amputation, a person may feel _____ in the missing limb.

9. A person with angina who experiences pain in the left arm is experiencing _____ pain.

10. During _____, needles are inserted to stimulate afferent neurons that inhibit pain signals.

D. Proprioceptors Inform Us of Our Position

Equilibrium	Muscle spindles	Vestibule	Golgi tendon organs
Proprioceptors	Ligaments	Semicircular	

1. _____ help us maintain the position of the body and its parts.

2. _____ are proprioceptors that detect movement.

3. _____ are proprioceptors that determine stretch in the tendons that attach muscle to bone.

4. Joint receptors detect movement in _____.

5. The brain coordinates information from proprioceptors with input from the _____

    and _____ canals in the inner ear to maintain _____ and coordination of muscular activities.

CHAPTER TEST

Select the correct response.

1. A stimulus is
    a. any change in the internal environment of the body.
    b. another name for the olfactory sense.
    c. any change in the outside environment.
    d. both a and c.

2. Stimuli are detected through
    a. sensory receptors.
    b. transducers.
    c. stimulus receivers.
    d. sensory detectors.

3. A(n) _____ would not be detected by a sensory receptor.
    a. idea

    b. mosquito bite
    c. sunset
    d. taste of a hot-fudge sundae

4. _____ help(s) to protect the eye anteriorly from foreign objects.
    a. Eyelashes
    b. Vitreous humor
    c. Retina
    d. Extrinsic muscles

5. _____ is not one of the layers of tissue that form the eyeball.
    a. Fibrous sclera
    b. Pinna
    c. Retina
    d. Choroid layer

6. The _____ is called the white of the eye.

a. cornea
b. sclera
c. retina
d. iris

7. The _____ is the colored part of the eye and can appear as blue, green, or brown.
   a. cornea
   b. sclera
   c. retina
   d. iris

8. The _____ is the transparent layer that covers the iris and the pupil at the front of the eye.
   a. cornea
   b. sclera
   c. retina
   d. lens

9. The _____ regulates the amount of light entering the eye.
   a. cornea
   b. sclera
   c. retina
   d. iris

10. The _____ contains sensory receptors called rods and cones.
    a. cornea
    b. sclera
    c. retina
    d. conjunctiva

11. The cones are responsible for
    a. night vision.
    b. color vision.
    c. day vision.
    d. both b and c.

12. The rods are responsible for
    a. night vision.
    b. color vision.
    c. day vision.
    d. both b and c.

13. The _____ is not an ossicle.
    a. malleus
    b. eustachian
    c. incus
    d. stapes

14. The _____ is a snail-shaped portion of the inner ear that contains the organ of Corti, the sound

receptors.
    a. perilymph
    b. bony labyrinth
    c. cochlea
    d. utricle

15. Hair cells in the organ of Corti
    a. are equipped with tiny projections called flagella.
    b. are equipped with tiny projections called stereocilia.
    c. filter out impurities entering the ear to protect the tympanic membrane.
    d. grow long and need to be cut periodically.

16. Although it varies to some degree, the human ear is generally equipped to register sound frequencies in the range of
    a. 1000 to 4000 Hz.
    b. 20 to 20,000 KHz.
    c. 20 to 20,000 Hz.
    d. 1000 to 4000 KHz.

17. The response of the sensory cells in the semicircular canals is produced by the flow of _____ within the canals as the position of the head changes.
    a. polylymph
    b. endolymph
    c. perilymph
    d. otoliths

18. The odors detected by the olfactory epithelium are transmitted by the
    a. olfactory nerve.
    b. auditory nerve.
    c. vestibular nerve.
    d. trigeminal nerve.

19. Sweet and salty tastes are sensed mainly
    a. at the tip of the tongue.
    b. at the sides of the tongue.
    c. at the posterior of the tongue.
    d. under the tongue.

20. Sour taste is detected mainly
    a. at the tip of the tongue.
    b. at the sides of the tongue.
    c. at the posterior of the tongue.
    d. under the tongue.

21. Bitter taste is detected mainly
    a.   at the tip of the tongue.
    b.   at the sides of the tongue.
    c.   at the posterior of the tongue.
    d.   under the tongue.

22. Thermoreceptors are especially concentrated in the
    a.   fingertips and toes.
    b.   scalp.
    c.   lips and mouth.
    d.   auditory canal.

23. When stimulated, nociceptors in the skin

transmit signals through sensory neurons to interneurons in the
    a.   motor cortex.
    b.   spinal cord.
    c.   visual cortex.
    d.   auditory canal.

24. Opiates work by blocking the release of
    a.   substance P.
    b.   acetylcholine.
    c.   gluconate.
    d.   endorphins.

25. Which is not a type of proprioceptor?
    a.   muscle spindles
    b.   endorphins
    c.   Golgi tendon organs
    d.   joint receptors

Chapter

9

ENDOCRINE CONTROL

■ ■ ■

Outline

Introduction
I. Many tissues secrete hormones or hormone-like substances.
II. Hormones combine with specific receptors on or in target cells.
   A. Many hormones act through second messengers and steroid hormones activate genes.
III. Hormone secretion is regulated by negative feedback mechanisms.
IV. The hypothalamus regulates the pituitary gland.
   A. The posterior lobe releases two hormones produced by the hypothalamus.
   B. The anterior lobe regulates growth and other endocrine glands.

   1. Growth hormone stimulates protein synthesis.
V. Thyroid hormones increase metabolic rate.
VI. Parathyroid glands regulate calcium concentration.
VII. The islets of Langerhans regulate glucose concentration.
   A. In diabetes mellitus, glucose accumulates in the blood.
VIII. The adrenal glands function in metabolism and stress.
   A. The adrenal medulla secretes epinephrine and norepinephrine.
   B. The adrenal cortex secretes steroid hormones.
   C. Stress threatens homeostasis.

Learning Objectives

After you have studied this chapter, you should be able to:

1. Describe the sources, transport, and general functions of hormones and hormone-like substances (neurohormones and prostaglandins).
2. Compare the mechanisms of action of hormones that work through second messengers and steroid hormones.
3. Describe how endocrine glands are regulated by negative feedback mechanisms.
4. Identify the principal endocrine glands, locate them in the body, and list the hormones secreted by each gland.
5. Justify describing the hypothalamus as the link between nervous and endocrine systems. (Describe the mechanisms by which the hypothalamus exerts its control.)

6. Compare the functions of the posterior and anterior lobes of the pituitary and describe the actions of their hormones.
7. Summarize the actions of the thyroid hormones and draw a diagram illustrating how they are regulated.
8. Describe how the parathyroid and thyroid glands regulate calcium levels.
9. Contrast the actions of insulin and glucagon and describe the effects of diabetes mellitus.
10. Describe the role of the adrenal medulla in the body's responses to stress.
11. Identify the hormones secreted by the adrenal cortex, and give the actions of glucocorticoids and mineralocorticoids.

STUDY QUESTIONS

Within each category, fill in the blanks with the correct response.

INTRODUCTION

Cells	Exocrine	Homeostasis	Reproduction	Endocrine	Fluid
Hormones	Target	Endocrinology	Growth	Metabolic	

1. The endocrine system helps regulate _____, _____, use of

   nutrients by _____, salt and _____ balance, and

   _____ rate.

2. _____ is the study of the endocrine system.

3. The endocrine system consists of specialized tissues and _____ glands which secrete

   chemical messengers called _____.

4. While _____ glands release their secretions into ducts, endocrine glands don't have
   ducts. They release their hormones into the surrounding interstitial fluid or blood.

5. _____ cells, the cells influenced by a particular hormone, may be located in another
   endocrine gland or in an entirely different type of organ.

6. The endocrine system works with the nervous system to maintain _____, or steady
   state of the body.

I. MANY TISSUES SECRETE HORMONES OR HORMONE-LIKE SUBSTANCES

Blood   Neuroendocrine   Prostaglandins   Hormones   Neurohormones

1. Certain neurons, known as _____ cells, are an important link between the nervous
   and endocrine systems.

2. Neuroendocrine cells produce _____ that are transported down axons and released
   into the interstitial fluid.

3. Neurohormones typically diffuse into capillaries and are transported by the _____.

4. _____ are a group of about 16 closely related lipids that are manufactured by many
   different tissues in the body.

5. Prostaglandins interact with other _____ to regulate various metabolic activities.

II.   HORMONES COMBINE WITH SPECIFIC RECEPTORS ON OR IN TARGET CELLS

First messenger   Receptors   Target

1.   A hormone may pass through many tissues "unnoticed" until it reaches its _____ cells.

2.   Target cells use specialized proteins on or in the cell to recognize a specific hormone. These proteins act as

_____ and bind the hormone.

3.   A hormone is referred to as a _____ because it initiates a series of reactions when it combines with a receptor.

A.   Many Hormones Act Through Second Messengers and Steroid Hormones Activate Genes

Calcium   Cyclic AMP   Second messenger   Calmodulin   Plasma   Steroid

1.   Hormones that are large molecules combine with receptors on the _____ membrane of the target cell.

2.   A hormone acting as a first messenger relays information to a _____ which may alter the activity of a cell.

3.   _____ ions can act as second messengers.

4.   Calcium ions bind to the protein _____.

5.   _____, or cAMP, is another second messenger.

6.   _____ hormones and thyroid hormones are relatively small molecules that pass easily through the plasma membrane of a target cell.

III.   HORMONE SECRETION IS REGULATED BY NEGATIVE FEEDBACK MECHANISMS

Endocrine gland   Hypersecretion   Negative feedback
Homeostasis   Hyposecretion   Parathyroid

1.   _____ depends on normal concentrations of hormones.

2.   Hormone secretion is typically regulated by _____ mechanisms.

3.   Information about the amount of hormone or of some other substance in the blood or interstitial fluid is fed

back to the _____ which then responds to restore homeostasis.

4.   The _____ glands regulate the calcium concentration of the blood.

5. In _____, the endocrine gland decreases its hormone output to abnormally low levels.

6. In _____, the endocrine gland increases its output to abnormally high levels, over-stimulating target cells.

IV. THE HYPOTHALAMUS REGULATES THE PITUITARY GLAND

Anterior   Hypothalamus   Pituitary gland   Releasing   Endocrine   Inhibiting   Posterior

1. The _____ links the nervous and endocrine systems.

2. Directly or indirectly, the hypothalamus regulates most _____ activity.

3. Oxytocin is a neurohormone which is stored in the _____.

4. _____ hormones and _____ hormones act on the pituitary gland, regulating secretion of several pituitary hormones.

5. The pituitary gland consists of two main lobes, the _____ lobe and the

_____ lobe.

A. The Posterior Lobe Releases Two Hormones Produced by the Hypothalamus

Antidiuretic hormone (ADH)   Inhibits   Oxytocin   Diabetes insipidus   Labor   Posterior lobe

1. The _____ of the pituitary gland secretes two hormones—oxytocin and antidiuretic hormone (ADH).

2. _____ stimulates contraction of smooth muscle in the wall of the uterus and stimulates release of milk from the breast.

3. Oxytocin is sometimes administered clinically to initiate or speed _____.

4. _____ regulates fluid balance in the body and indirectly helps control blood pressure.

5. Alcohol consumption increases urine output because alcohol _____ ADH secretion.

6. ADH deficiency can lead to the condition known as _____, in which enormous quantities of urine may be excreted.

B. The Anterior Lobe Regulates Growth and Other Endocrine Glands

| Adrenal cortex | Inhibiting | Releasing | Anterior lobe | |
| Portal | Thyroid | Gonadotropic | Prolactin | Tropic |

1. The _____ of the pituitary gland secretes growth hormone, prolactin, and several other hormones that stimulate other endocrine glands.

2. A _____ hormone stimulates other endocrine glands.

3. Each of the anterior pituitary hormones is regulated in some way by a(n) _____

    hormone, and in some cases by a(n) _____ hormone produced in the hypothalamus.

4. _____ veins are unusual in that they do not deliver blood to a larger vein directly, but connect two sets of capillaries.

5. During lactation, _____ stimulates the cells of the mammary glands to secrete milk.

6. TSH stimulates the _____ gland.

7. ACTH stimulates the _____.

8. Follicle stimulating hormone and luteinizing hormone are _____ hormones.

1. Growth Hormone Stimulates Protein Synthesis

| Growth hormone | Pulses | Hypothalamus | Pituitary | Insulin-like growth factors |
| Sex | Increases | Somatomedins | Psychosocial dwarfism | |

1. _____ stimulates body growth mainly by stimulating protein synthesis.

2. Growth hormone (GH) stimulates liver cells and cells of many other tissues to produce peptides called

    _____, including _____.

3. A high level of growth hormone in the blood signals the _____ to secrete the

    inhibiting hormone, and the _____ release of growth hormone slows.

4. Secretion of growth hormone _____ during exercise.

5. Growth hormone is released in a series of _____ 2 to 4 hours after a meal.

6. In extreme cases, childhood stress can produce a form of retarded development known as

    _____.

7. _____ hormones must be present for the adolescent growth spurt to occur.

V. THYROID HORMONES INCREASE METABOLIC RATE

Goiter	Hypothyroidism	Thyroid gland	Hypersecretion	Negative feedback system
T_3	Thyroid hormones	Thyroxine	Hyposecretion	Thyroid-stimulating hormone

1. The _____ is shaped somewhat like a shield and is located in the neck.

2. The _____ are essential for normal growth and development and they increase metabolic rate in most tissues.

3. The main thyroid hormone is _____, or T_4.

4. A second thyroid hormone _____, or triiodothyronine, has three iodine atoms in its structure.

5. The regulation of thyroid hormone secretion depends on a _____ between the anterior pituitary and the thyroid gland.

6. The anterior pituitary secretes _____, which promotes synthesis and secretion of thyroid hormones.

7. _____ during childhood results in low metabolic rate and retarded mental and physical development.

8. Any abnormal enlargement of the thyroid gland is termed a _____.

9. A goiter may be associated with either _____ or _____.

VI. PARATHYROID GLANDS REGULATE CALCIUM CONCENTRATION

Calcitonin   Increases   Parathyroid hormones   Calcium   Parathyroid glands   Vitamin D

1. The _____ are embedded in the connective tissue that surrounds the thyroid gland.

2. The parathyroid glands secrete _____, a small protein that regulates the calcium level of the blood and tissue fluid.

3. Parathyroid hormone _____ calcium levels by stimulating release of calcium from the bones.

4. Parathyroid hormone also activates _____, which then increases the amount of calcium absorbed from the intestine.

5. The parathyroid glands are regulated by the concentration of _____ in the blood and tissue fluid.

6. When calcium concentration becomes very high, _____ is released from the thyroid gland.

VII.   THE ISLETS OF LANGERHANS REGULATE GLUCOSE CONCENTRATION

Alpha	Digestive	Glucagon	Insulin	Endocrine	Islets of Langerhans
Glucose	Opposite	Beta Cells	Antagonistically	Exocrine	Posterior

1. The pancreas lies in the abdomen just _____ to the stomach.

2. The pancreas has both _____ and _____ functions.

3. The exocrine cells of the pancreas produce _____ enzymes.

4. More than a million small clusters of cells known as the _____ are scattered through-
    out the pancreas.

5. About 70% of the islet cells are _____ that produce the hormone insulin.

6. _____ cells secrete the hormone glucagon.

7. _____ lowers the concentration of the glucose in the blood.

8. Insulin activity results in lowering the _____ level in the blood.

9. _____ raises the blood glucose level by stimulating liver cells to convert glycogen to
    glucose.

10. The effects of glucagon are _____ to those of insulin.

11. Insulin and glucagon work _____ to keep blood glucose concentration within
    normal limits.

A.   In Diabetes Mellitus, Glucose Accumulates in the Blood

Diabetes mellitus   Insulin resistance   Type 2   Insulin   Type 1   Urine

1. The main disorder associated with pancreatic hormones is _____.

2. Insulin-dependent diabetes, referred to as _____ diabetes, usually develops before age
    20.

3. Type 1 diabetes is clinically treated with _____.

4. About 90% of all cases of diabetes are non-insulin–dependent, or _____ diabetes.

5. In type 2 diabetes, insulin receptors on target cells are not able to bind with the insulin and use it. This

    condition is known as _____.

6. In diabetics, blood glucose concentration may be so high that glucose is excreted in the

_____.

VIII. THE ADRENAL GLANDS FUNCTION IN METABOLISM AND STRESS

Adrenal cortex   Adrenal medulla   Stress   Adrenal glands   Metabolism

1. The paired _____ are small, yellow masses of tissue located above the kidneys.

2. Each adrenal gland consists of a central portion known as the _____, and a larger

   outer region, the _____.

3. Both regions of the adrenal glands function as distinct glands. Both secrete hormones that help regulate

   _____, and both help the body deal with _____.

A. The Adrenal Medulla Secretes Epinephrine and Norepinephrine

Adrenal medulla   Emergency   Metabolic   Neurotransmitter
Dilate   Epinephrine   Norepinephrine

1. The _____ develops from nervous tissue and is sometimes considered part of the
   sympathetic nervous system.

2. The adrenal medulla secretes two hormones: _____ and

   _____.

3. Norepinephrine is the same substance that is secreted as a _____ by sympathetic
   neurons and by some neurons in the central nervous system.

4. The adrenal medulla is the _____ gland of the body because it prepares us to deal
   with threatening situations.

5. Epinephrine and norepinephrine can increase the _____ rate as much as 100%.

6. Epinephrine and norepinephrine can _____ the airways so that breathing is more
   effective.

B. The Adrenal Cortex Secretes Steroid Hormones

Adrenal cortex   Estrogen   Glucose   Corticotropin releasing factor
Mineralocorticoids   Aldosterone   Potassium   Adrenocorticotropic hormone
Glucocorticoids   Cortisol   Sodium   Androgen

1. The _____ secretes three different types of steroid hormones.

2. _____ help the body cope with stress.

3. The main glucocorticoid is _____, also called hydrocortisone.

4. The principal action of the glucocorticoids is to promote production of _____ from other nutrients.

5. _____ regulate water and salt balance.

6. _____ is the principal mineralocorticoid.

7. The main function of aldosterone is to maintain homeostasis of _____ and

   _____ ions.

8. The sex hormones, _____ and _____ are secreted by the adrenal cortex in minute amounts in both sexes.

9. Stress stimulates the hypothalamus to secrete _____, or CRF.

10. CRF stimulates the anterior pituitary to secrete _____, or ACTH.

C.   Stress Threatens Homeostasis

Adrenal   Homeostasis   Norepinephrine   Sympathetic   Epinephrine   Hormones   Stressors

1. Good health and survival depend on maintaining _____.

2. _____ are stimuli that disrupt the steady state of the body.

3. During a stress response, the brain sends messages activating the _____ nervous

   system and the _____ glands.

4. When the body is reacting to stress, the hormones _____ and

   _____ are released, and the body prepares for fight or flight.

5. Chronic stress is harmful because of the effects of long-term elevation of some

   _____.

Labeling Exercise

Please fill in the correct labels for Figure 9-1.

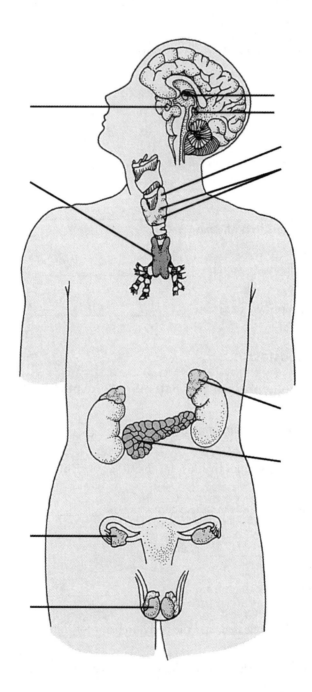

Figure 9-1

CHAPTER TEST

Select the correct response.

1. The _____ system works with the nervous system to maintain the steady state of the body.
   a. circulatory
   b. digestive
   c. endocrine
   d. reproductive

2. The endocrine system helps regulate
   a. growth.
   b. reproduction.
   c. metabolic rate.
   d. all of the above.

3. The endocrine system consists of tissues and glands that secrete chemical messengers called
   a. hormones.
   b. receptors.
   c. chemical secretors.
   d. capillaries.

4. Hormones act on cells referred to as
   a. alpha cells.
   b. target cells.
   c. hormonal cells.
   d. glandular cells.

5. _____ are a group of closely related lipids that are manufactured by many different tissues in the body.
   a. Hormones
   b. Phospholipids
   c. Prostaglandins
   d. Glandular lipids

6. Prostaglandins are manufactured in the
   a. prostate gland.
   b. lungs.
   c. liver.
   d. all of the above.

7. At present, prostaglandins are used to
   a. induce labor.
   b. cure multiple sclerosis.
   c. treat chronic bronchitis.
   d. retard the AIDS virus

8. Most endocrine activity is regulated by the
   a. hypothalamus.
   b. hyperthalamus.
   c. thyroid.
   d. target cells.

9. The _____ gland is sometimes called the master gland of the body.
   a. thyroid
   b. pituitary
   c. lymph
   d. endocrine

10. The hormone _____ stimulates contraction of smooth muscle in the wall of the uterus.
    a. ADH
    b. ACTH
    c. oxytocin
    d. somatropin

11. _____ regulates fluid balance in the body and indirectly helps control blood pressure.
    a. ADH
    b. ACTH
    c. Oxytocin
    d. Somatropin

12. ADH deficiency leads to the condition called _____, in which enormous quantities of urine may be excreted.
    a. diabetes mellitus
    b. diabetes insipidus
    c. type 1 diabetes
    d. type 2 diabetes

13. The main thyroid hormone is
    a. ADH.
    b. ACTH.
    c. oxytocin.
    d. thyroxine.

14. Beta cells produce the hormone
    a. glucagon.
    b. ADH.
    c. insulin.
    d. oxytocin.

15. Alpha cells produce the hormone
    a. glucagon.
    b. ADH.
    c. insulin.
    d. oxytocin.

16. The main disorder associated with pancreatic hormones is
    a. diabetes insipidus.
    b. diabetes mellitus.
    c. pancreatic cancer.
    d. dwarfism.

17. The normal fasting blood glucose level is about
    a. 10 mg/dl.
    b. 90 mg/dl.
    c. 300 mg/dl.
    d. 1000 mg/dl.

18. Which of the following are actions of epineph-
    rine and norepinephrine?
    a. increase metabolic rate by as much as 100%
    b. a weakening of muscle contraction
    c. increase blood pressure
    d. a and c

19. Which of the following are stressors?
    a. being sick
    b. taking a test
    c. getting married
    d. all of the above

CROSSWORD PUZZLE FOR CHAPTERS 6, 7, 8, AND 9

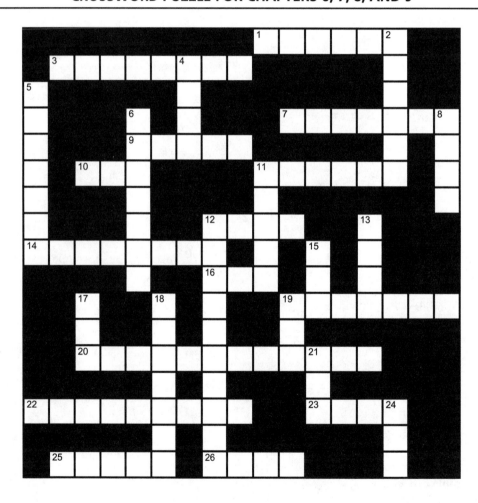

Across

1. Region of spinal cord below the thoracic level
3. Part of the brain that controls voluntary movement
7. Part of the brain that regulates heart rate and blood pressure
9. Second cranial nerve
10. Part of nervous system consisting of brain and spinal cord
11. Gray matter of cerebrum
12. Part of the brain that helps regulate respiration
14. Transmits impulses to cell body
16. An action system of the brain
19. Nerve that supplies the diaphragm
20. Part of the brain that controls body temperature
22. Releases growth hormone
23. Outer layer of the meninges
25. Opening through which light enters the eye
26. Focuses light on retina

Down

2. Automatic sequence of stimulus response
4. Sensory fibers enter the spinal cord through the dorsal _____
5. Gland that stimulates metabolic rate
6. Controlled by the cerebellum
8. Transmits impulses from the cell body toward the synapse
11. Sensitive to color
12. Part of the nervous system that includes sense organs
13. Each of the six divisions of the cerebral hemisphere is called a _____
15. Hormone that regulates calcium level
17. Tropic hormone released by anterior pituitary gland
18. Lobe where Broca's speech area is located
19. Innermost of the three meninges
21. Visual and auditory reflex centers are located in the _____ brain
24. Hormone that stimulates reabsorption of water

Chapter

10

THE CIRCULATORY SYSTEM: BLOOD

■ ■ ■

Outline

Introduction
I. Plasma is the fluid component of blood.
II. Red blood cells transport oxygen.
III. White blood cells defend the body against disease.
IV. Platelets function in blood clotting.

V. Successful blood transfusions depend on blood groups.
   A. The ABO blood groups are based on antigens A and B.
   B. The Rh system consists of several Rh antigens.

Learning Objectives

After you have studied this chapter, you should be able to:

1. Describe the subsystems, components, and functions of the circulatory system.
2. Describe the composition of blood plasma and the functions of plasma proteins.
3. Relate the structure and function of red blood cells; summarize the red blood cell life cycle.
4. Compare the structure and functions of the various types of white blood cells.

5. Describe the structure and function of platelets and summarize the chemical events of blood clotting.
6. Identify the antigen and antibody associated with each ABO blood type and explain why blood types must be carefully matched in transfusion therapy.
7. Identify the cause and importance of Rh incompatibility.

STUDY QUESTIONS

Within each category, fill in the blanks with the correct response.

INTRODUCTION

Blood   Disease   Lymphatic   Cardiovascular   Fluid   Plasma   Circulatory   Heart   Platelets

1. The _____ system is the transportation system of the body.

2. The circulatory system consists of two subsystems: the _____ system and the

   _____ system.

3. In the cardiovascular system, the _____ pumps blood through a vast system of blood vessels.

4. As it circulates, the _____ transports nutrients, oxygen, hormones, and waste products.

5. The lymphatic system helps preserve _____ balance and protects the body against

_____.

6. Blood consists of red blood cells, white blood cells, and cell fragments called _____,

all suspended in a yellowish fluid called _____.

I. PLASMA IS THE FLUID COMPONENT OF BLOOD

Acid-base	**Gamma**	**pH**	**Globulins**	**Plasma proteins**	**Alpha globulins**
Albumins	**Prothrombin**	**Beta**	**Serum**	**Interstitial fluid**	
Fibrinogen	**Liver**	**Water**	**Intracellular fluid**		

1. Plasma consists mainly of _____.

2. Plasma is in dynamic equilibrium with the _____ bathing the cells and with the

_____ inside cells.

3. Plasma contains several kinds of _____, each with specific properties and functions.

4. Most plasma proteins are manufactured in the _____.

5. Plasma proteins may be divided into three groups, or fractions: _____,

_____, and _____.

6. Plasma proteins are important _____ buffers, and help keep the

_____ of the blood within a narrow homeostatic range.

7. _____ include certain hormones and proteins that transport hormones.

8. _____ is an alpha globulin involved in blood clotting.

9. _____ globulins include lipoproteins that transport fats and cholesterol, as well as proteins that transport certain vitamins and minerals.

10. The _____ globulin fraction contains many types of antibodies that provide immunity to diseases such as measles and infectious hepatitis.

11. When the proteins involved in clotting have been removed from the plasma, the remaining liquid is called

_____ .

II. RED BLOOD CELLS TRANSPORT OXYGEN

Anemia	Iron deficiency	Oxygen	Biconcave	Kidneys	Oxyhemoglobin
Marrow	Erythropoietin	Hemoglobin	Nucleus	Stem cells	Red blood cells

1. _____ are one of the most specialized cell types in the body.

2. Red blood cells are adapted for producing and packaging _____, the red pigment that transports oxygen.

3. A mature red blood cell is a tiny, flexible, _____ disk, which provides for a high ratio of surface area to volume, allowing efficient diffusion of _____ and carbon dioxide into and out of the cell.

4. A mature red blood cell lacks a _____ and most other organelles.

5. As blood flows through the lungs, oxygen combines weakly with hemoglobin to form

_____ .

6. In children, red blood cells are produced in the red bone _____ of almost all bones.

7. Red bone marrow has immature cells known as _____ .

8. Red blood cell production is regulated by the hormone _____ .

9. Erythropoietin is secreted by the _____ in response to a decrease in oxygen concentration.

10. A hemoglobin deficiency is called _____ .

11. _____ is the most common cause of anemia.

III. WHITE BLOOD CELLS DEFEND THE BODY AGAINST DISEASE

Enzymes	Neutrophils	Antibodies	Lymphocytes	Parasitic
Attack	Granular	Phagocytes	Macrophages	Phagocytosis
Basophils	Histamine	Lysosomes	Monocytes	Tissues
Heparin	Eosinophils	Bacteria	Leukocytes	Allergic reactions

1. White blood cells, or _____, are specialized to protect the body against harmful bacteria and other microorganisms that cause disease.

2. Whereas red blood cells function within the blood, many white cells leave the circulation and perform their duties in various _____.

3. _____ is the process by which cells engulf microorganisms, foreign particles, or other cells.

4. _____ are cells that are specialized to carry on phagocytosis.

5. _____ leukocytes have large, lobed nuclei and distinctive granules in their cytoplasm.

6. The kinds of white blood cells that contain granules are _____,

    _____, and _____.

7. Neutrophils are adept at seeking out and ingesting _____.

8. Most of the granules in neutrophils contain _____ that digest ingested material.

9. The _____ of eosinophils contain enzymes such as oxidases.

10. Eosinophils increase in number during _____, and during

     _____ infestations.

11. Granules in the cytoplasm of basophils contain _____, a substance that dilates blood vessels and makes capillaries more permeable.

12. Other basophil granules contain _____, an anticoagulant that helps prevent blood from clotting inappropriately within the blood vessels.

13. Two types of agranular white blood cells are _____ and

     _____.

14. Some lymphocytes are specialized to make _____, others

     _____ bacteria.

15. Monocytes migrate into the connective tissues and develop into _____, the large scavenger cells of the body.

IV.   PLATELETS FUNCTION IN BLOOD CLOTTING

Liver	**Thrombocytes**	**Fibrin**	**Thrombin**	**Platelet plug**	**Prothrombin activator**
Serum	**Vitamin K**	**Fibrinogen**	**Prevent**	**Clotting factors**	

1. Platelets, also called _____, are tiny fragments of cytoplasm that become detached from certain very large cells in the bone marrow.

2. Platelets _____ blood loss.

3. When a blood vessel is cut, platelets stick to the rough, cut edges of the blood vessel, forming a

   _____ that seals the hole in the blood vessel wall.

4. During the clotting process, platelets and injured tissue release substances that activate

   _____ in the blood. A series of reactions takes place that results in formation of an

   enzyme known as _____.

5. Prothrombin activator catalyzes the conversion of prothrombin to its active form,

   _____.

6. Prothrombin is manufactured in the _____ with the help of

   _____.

7. Thrombin acts as an enzyme that converts the plasma protein _____ to fibrin.

8. _____ threads form the webbing of a blood clot.

9. As a blood clot contracts, it squeezes out _____.

V.   SUCCESSFUL BLOOD TRANSFUSIONS DEPEND ON BLOOD GROUPS

Agglutinate	**Donors**	**Recipients**	**Antibodies**	**Hemolysis**
Centrifuge	**Whole**	**Plasma**	**Transfusions**	**Transfusion reaction**

1. Blood _____—the transfer of blood from healthy _____ to

   _____ in need of blood—are routine, lifesaving procedures.

2. Blood components can be separated by a _____.

3. _____ can be used to expand blood volume in patients who are in circulatory shock.

4. _____ blood, or blood components, can be stored in blood banks and withdrawn as needed.

5. If blood is not carefully matched before a transfusion, a _____ may occur.

6. During a transfusion reaction, _____ in the recipient's blood attack the foreign red blood cells in the transfused blood, causing them to _____ or clump.

7. _____ occurs when red blood cells break, releasing hemoglobin into the plasma.

A. The ABO Blood Groups Are Based on Antigens A and B

Anti-A	**Antigens**	**Universal donors**	**Anti-B**
Repeated	**Antibodies**	**Universal recipients**	**Type O**

1. Red blood cells have specific proteins called _____ on their cell surfaces.

2. Individuals with type O blood have neither type of antigen on their red cells, and are referred to as

_____ because they can donate blood to patients with any blood type.

3. Certain _____ called agglutinins are found in the plasma.

4. People with type A blood have _____ antibodies circulating in their blood.

5. People with Type B blood have _____ antibodies circulating in their blood.

6. People with _____ blood have both anti-A and anti-B antibodies in their blood.

7. Blood mismatching can be fatal, especially if the mistake is ever _____.

8. _____ have type AB blood and don't have antibodies to either type A or type B blood.

B. The Rh System Consists of Several Rh Antigens

Antigen D	**Red blood cells**	**Exposed**	**Rh antigens**	**Rh incompatibility**
Rh negative	**Hemolytic anemia**	**Rh factor**	**Rh positive**	

1. The Rh system consists of more then 40 kinds of _____.

2. Each Rh antigen is referred to as an _____.

3. The most important Rh factor is _____.

4. Most persons of western European descent are _____, which means that they have

    antigen D on the surfaces of their _____.

5. The approximately 15% of the population who are _____ have no antigen D on
    their red blood cell surfaces.

6. Antibody D does not occur in the blood of Rh negative persons unless they have been

    _____ to antigen D.

7. Although several kinds of maternal-fetal blood type incompatibilities are known,

    _____ is probably the most important.

8. The condition known as _____ occurs in a fetus or newborn when the mother's Rh
    positive antibodies cross the placenta and cause hemolysis of the baby's red blood cells.

CHAPTER TEST

Select the correct response.

1. The circulatory system does all of the following
    except
    a. transport nutrients from the digestive system
        to all parts of the body.
    b. move voluntary skeletal muscles.
    c. transport carbon dioxide and other meta-
        bolic wastes from the cells to the excretory
        organs.
    d. transport oxygen from the lungs to all of the
        cells of the body.

2. The circulatory system consists of the
    a. cardiovascular system.
    b. endocrine system.
    c. lymphatic system.
    d. a and c only.

3. Blood consists of
    a. red blood cells.
    b. white blood cells.
    c. platelets.
    d. all of the above.

4. Plasma consists of
    a. salt.
    b. water.
    c. proteins.
    d. all of the above.

5. The _____ serve as antibodies, which provide
    immunity against disease.
    a. gamma globulins
    b. fibrinogens
    c. albumins
    d. beta globulins

6. Fibrinogen is manufactured in the
    a. liver.
    b. lymph tissues.
    c. lungs.
    d. spleen.

7. _____ are adapted for producing and packaging
    hemoglobin.
    a. Red blood cells
    b. White blood cells
    c. Eosinophils
    d. Leukocytes

8. Red blood cells are produced in
    a. bone tissue.
    b. muscle tissue.
    c. red bone marrow.
    d. all bone marrow.

9. _____ defend the body against agents that cause disease.
   a. White blood cells
   b. Red blood cells
   c. Leukocytes
   d. Both a and c

10. The three types of white blood cells that contain granules are
    a. neutrophils, monocytes, and lymphocytes.
    b. basophils, eosinophils, and neutrophils.
    c. eosinophils, basophils, and lymphocytes.
    d. neutrophils, basophils, and monocytes.

11. The two types of white blood cells that lack specific granules in their cytoplasm are
    a. neutrophils and lymphocytes.
    b. neutrophils and monocytes.
    c. lymphocytes and monocytes.
    d. basophils and monocytes.

12. Prothrombin is a globulin found in plasma; it is manufactured in the _____ with the help of vitamin K.
    a. liver
    b. spleen
    c. stomach
    d. kidneys

13. Individuals with type AB blood have _____ antigens on their red blood cells.
    a. A
    b. B
    c. both A and B
    d. none of the above

14. Individuals with type O blood have _____ antigens on their red blood cells.
    a. A
    b. B
    c. both A and B
    d. none of the above

15. The most important of the Rh factors is
    a. antigen R.
    b. antigen D.
    c. Rh negative.
    d. Rh positive.

Chapter

11

THE CIRCULATORY SYSTEM: THE HEART

■ ■ ■

Outline

Introduction
I. The heart wall consists of three layers.
II. The heart has four chambers.
III. Valves prevent backflow of blood.
IV. The heart has its own blood vessels.
V. The conduction system consists of specialized cardiac muscles.
VI. The cardiac cycle includes contraction and relaxation phases.
VII. Closure of the valves causes the heart sounds.
VIII. Cardiac output varies with the body's needs.
IX. The heart is regulated by the nervous and endocrine systems.

Learning Objectives

After you have studied this chapter, you should be able to:

1. Describe the structure of the wall of the heart.
2. Identify the chambers of the heart and compare their functions.
3. Locate the atrioventricular and semilunar valves and compare their structure.
4. Identify the principal blood vessels that serve the heart wall.
5. Trace the path of an electrical impulse through the conduction system of the heart.
6. Describe the events of the cardiac cycle and correlate them with normal heart sounds.
7. Identify factors that influence cardiac output and explain how the heart is regulated.

STUDY QUESTIONS

Within each category, fill in the blanks with the correct response.

INTRODUCTION

Blood   Midline   Organ   Thorax

1. The heart is a hollow, muscular _____ not much bigger than a fist.

2. Depending on the body's changing needs, the heart can vary its output form 5 to 35 liters of

   _____ per minute.

3. The heart is located in the _____ between the lungs.

4. About two-thirds of the heart lies to the left of the body's _____.

I. THE HEART WALL CONSISTS OF THREE LAYERS

Blood	**Epicardium**	**Pericardium**	**Cardiac**	**Heart**	**Pericardial cavity**
Lymph	**Endocardium**	**Parietal**	**Endothelial**	**Visceral**	**Myocardium**

1. The wall of the _____ is richly supplied with nerves, _____

   vessels, and _____ vessels.

2. From the inside out, the layers of the heart are the _____,

   _____, and _____.

3. The endocardium consists of a smooth _____ lining resting on connective tissue.

4. The greatest bulk of the heart wall consists of the myocardium, the _____ muscle
   that contracts to pump the blood.

5. The outer layer of the heart is the _____, or _____ pericardium.

6. The pericardium consists of two layers that are separated by a potential space, the

   _____.

7. The outer layer of the pericardium, the _____ pericardium, forms a strong sac for
   the heart and helps to anchor it within the thorax.

II. THE HEART HAS FOUR CHAMBERS

Atria Heart Interventricular Septum Auricle Interatrial Pulmonary Ventricles

1. The _____ is a double pump.

2. The right and left sides of the heart are completely separated by a wall, or _____.

3. The _____ receive blood returning to the heart from the veins and act as reservoirs
   between contractions of the heart.

4. The _____ pump blood into the great arteries leaving the heart.

5. _____ arteries carry blood to the lungs, where gases are exchanged.

6. The wall between the atria is the _____ septum.

7. The wall between the ventricles is the _____ septum.

8. A small muscular pouch called the _____ increases the surface area of each atrium.

Labeling Exercise

Please fill in the correct labels for Figure 11-1.

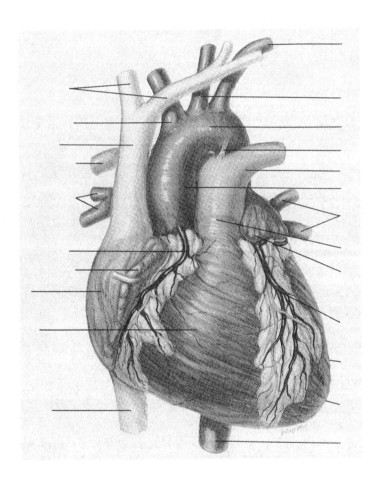

Figure 11-1

III. VALVES PREVENT BACKFLOW OF BLOOD

Aortic	Cusps	Pulmonary	Atrioventricular	Mitral
Semilunar	Bicuspid	Mitral stenosis	Tricuspid	

1. To prevent blood from flowing backward into the atrium, a(n) _____ valve guards the passageway between each atrium and ventricle.

2. The atrioventricular valve consists of flaps or _____ of fibrous tissues that project from the heart wall.

3. The atrioventricular valve between the right atrium and the right ventricle has three cusps and is called the

_____ valve.

4. The left atrioventricular valve, which has only two cusps, is called the _____ valve.

5. The bicuspid valve is commonly called the _____ valve.

6. A common valve deformity is _____, a narrowing of the opening of the mitral valve.

7. The _____ valves guard the exits from the ventricles.

8. The semilunar valve between the left ventricle and the aorta is called the _____ valve.

9. The semilunar valve between the right ventricle and the pulmonary artery is called the

_____ valve.

IV.   THE HEART HAS ITS OWN BLOOD VESSELS

Cardiac   **Coronary arteries**   **Coronary veins**   **Right atrium**
Coronary   **Coronary sinus**   **Oxygen**

1. The wall of the heart is so thick that _____ and nutrients are not able to effectively diffuse to all of its cells.

2. Blood vessels must deliver oxygen and nutrients to the _____ muscle in the heart wall.

3. Two _____ arteries branch off from the aorta as it leaves the heart.

4. Branches of the _____ bring blood to all the tissue of the heart.

5. Blood leaving the heart wall flows through _____.

6. The coronary veins join to form a large vein, the _____, which empties into the

_____.

V.   THE CONDUCTION SYSTEM CONSISTS OF SPECIALIZED CARDIAC MUSCLES

Atrioventricular   Conduction   Myocardium   Bundle   Intercalated   Sinoatrial

1. The heart has its own specialized _____ system and can beat independently from its nerve supply.

2. The _____ node is a small mass of specialized muscle in the posterior wall of the right atrium; it is called the pacemaker of the heart.

3. The _____ node, located in the right atrium along the lower part of the septum, delays the transmission of an impulse to allow the atria to complete their contraction before the ventricles contract.

4. From the atrioventricular node, a muscle impulse spreads into specialized muscle fibers that form the atrioventricular _____.

5. The ends of the fibers of the atrioventricular bundle connect to fibers of ordinary cardiac muscle within the _____.

6. Cardiac muscle fibers are joined at their ends by dense bands called _____ discs.

VI. THE CARDIAC CYCLE INCLUDES CONTRACTION AND RELAXATION PHASES

| **Arteries** | **Diastole** | **Systole** | **Atria** | **Electrocardiogram** |
| **Veins** | **Cardiac cycle** | **Semilunar** | **Ventricles** | |

1. The events that occur during one complete heartbeat make up the _____.

2. The period of contraction of the heart muscle is known as _____.

3. The period of relaxation of the heart muscle is called _____.

4. An electrical impulse is generated at the beginning of each cardiac cycle and spreads from the sinoatrial node

    throughout the _____.

5. As the atria contract, the atrioventricular valves open, and blood is forced from the atria into the

    _____.

6. As blood is forced from the atria into the ventricles, the _____ valves close.

7. As the atria relax, they are filled with blood from the _____.

8. As the ventricles contract, blood is forced through the semilunar valves into the

    _____.

9. The written record produced by using electrodes placed on the body surface on opposite sides of the heart to

    measure electrical activity in the heart is called a(n) _____.

VII. CLOSURE OF THE VALVES CAUSES THE HEART SOUNDS

Blood   Heart murmurs   Lub-dup   Valve   Diastole   Hissing   Stethoscope   Ventricular

1. When you listen to the heart through a _____, you can hear certain characteristic

    sounds, usually described as a _____.

2. The first sound, the "lub," marks the beginning of the _____ systole.

3. _____ is longer than systole, so when the heart is beating at a normal rate, there is a
    slight pause after the second sound.

4. Abnormal heart sounds called _____ indicate the possibility of valve disorders.

5. When a valve does not close properly, some _____ may flow backward, which may

    result in a _____ sound.

6. Murmurs can also be detected when a _____ becomes narrowed and rough.

VIII. CARDIAC OUTPUT VARIES WITH THE BODY'S NEEDS

Cardiac   Heart rate   Stroke volume   Ventricle   Cardiac output
Venous   Heart   Norepinephrine   Starling's

1. The _____ is the volume of blood pumped by the left ventricle into the aorta in one
    minute.

2. The volume of blood pumped by one ventricle during one beat is called the _____.

3. By multiplying the stroke volume by the number of times the left _____ beats per

    minute, the _____ output can be computed.

4. Cardiac output varies with changes in either stroke volume or _____.

5. The amount of blood delivered to the heart by the veins is _____ return.

6. According to _____ law of the _____, the greater the
    amount of blood delivered to the heart by the veins, the more blood the heart pumps.

7. The release of _____ by sympathetic nerves increases the force of contraction of the
    cardiac muscle fibers.

IX.   THE HEART IS REGULATED BY THE NERVOUS AND ENDOCRINE SYSTEMS

Acetylcholine	**Blood pressure**	**Decreases**	**Tachycardia**	**Autonomic**
Bradycardia	**Norepinephrine**	**Beta-adrenergic**	**Cardiac centers**	**SA**

1.   Sensory receptors in the walls of certain blood vessels and heart chambers are sensitive to changes in

     _____.

2.   When stimulated, sensory receptors send messages to _____ in the medulla of the
     brain.

3.   Cardiac centers in the medulla maintain control over two sets of _____ nerves that

     pass to the _____ node.

4.   Parasympathetic nerves release the neurotransmitter _____, which slows the heart.

5.   Sympathetic nerves release _____, which speeds the heart rate and increases the
     strength of contraction.

6.   Norepinephrine binds to receptors known as _____ receptors.

7.   A fast heart rate of over 100 beats per minute is called _____.

8.   A slow heart rate of less than 60 beats per minute is referred to as _____.

9.   Heart rate _____ when body temperature is lowered.

Labeling Exercise

Please fill in the correct labels for Figure 11-2.

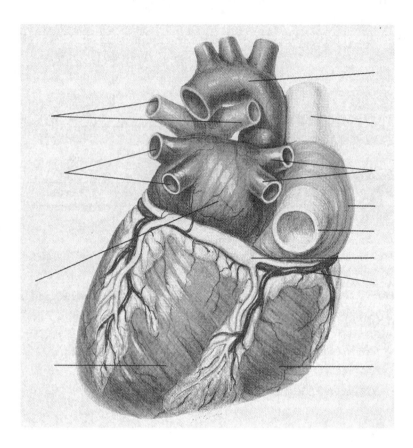

Figure 11-2

CHAPTER TEST

Select the correct response.

1. The wall of the heart is richly supplied with all but which of the following?
   a. nerves
   b. blood vessels
   c. skeletal muscle
   d. lymph vessels

2. From the inside out, the layers of the heart are
   a. endocardium, myocardium, and pericardium.
   b. myocardium, endocardium, and pericardium.
   c. pericardium, myocardium, and endocardium.
   d. pericardium, endocardium, and myocardium.

3. The inner layer, or _____ consists of a smooth endothelial lining that is resting on connective tissue.
   a. myocardium
   b. pericardium
   c. endocardium
   d. epicardium

4. The greatest portion of the heart wall consists of _____, the cardiac muscle that contracts to pump blood.
   a. myocardium
   b. pericardium
   c. endocardium
   d. epicardium

5. The outer layer of the heart is called the
    a. myocardium.
    b. pericardium.
    c. endocardium.
    d. b and c only.

6. The _____ receive blood returning to the heart
    from the veins and act as reservoirs between
    contractions of the heart.
    a. ventricles
    b. atria
    c. arteries
    d. septa

7. The _____ pump blood into the great arteries
    leaving the heart.
    a. ventricles
    b. atria
    c. capillaries
    d. septa

8. A small muscular pouch called an _____
    increases the surface area of each atrium.
    a. interatrial septum
    b. interventricular septum
    c. auricle
    d. atrial pouch

9. The atrioventricular valve between the right
    atrium and right ventricle is called the _____
    valve.
    a. tricuspid
    b. bicuspid
    c. mitral
    d. b and c only

10. The atrioventricular valve between the left
    atrium and the left ventricle is called the _____
    valve.
    a. tricuspid
    b. bicuspid
    c. mitral
    d. both b and c

11. The cusps of each _____ valve are shaped like
    half-moons.
    a. tricuspid
    b. bicuspid
    c. semilunar
    d. mitral

12. The semilunar valve between the left ventricle
    and the aorta is called the _____ valve.
    a. ventricular
    b. aortic
    c. pulmonary
    d. mitral

13. The semilunar valve between the right ventricle
    and the pulmonary artery is called the _____
    valve.
    a. ventricular
    b. aortic
    c. pulmonary
    d. mitral

14. Two _____ arteries branch off from the aorta as
    it leaves the heart.
    a. coronary
    b. pulmonary
    c. aortic
    d. sinoatrial

15. The heart's conduction system is made up of
    specialized _____ muscle.
    a. smooth
    b. cardiac
    c. pulmonary
    d. skeletal

16. The _____ is a small mass of specialized muscle
    in the posterior wall of the right atrium.
    a. atrioventricular node
    b. sinoatrial node
    c. sinoatrial bundle
    d. atrioventricular bundle

17. From the AV node, an electrical impulse spreads
    into specialized muscle fibers that form the
    a. atrioventricular bundle.
    b. cardiac bundle.
    c. sinoatrial bundle.
    d. sinoatrial node.

18. A cardiac cycle occurs approximately _____
    times per minute
    a. 7
    b. 25
    c. 72
    d. 150

19. The period of contraction is known as
    a. diastole.
    b. systole.
    c. fibrillation.
    d. asystole.

20. The period of relaxation is known as
    a. diastole.
    b. systole.
    c. fibrillation.
    d. asystole.

21. The written record produced by an electrocardiograph is called a(n)
    a. ECG.
    b. EKG.
    c. electrocardiogram.
    d. all of the above.

22. Abnormal heart sounds are called
    a. heart mumbles.
    b. valve stenosis.
    c. heart murmurs.
    d. valve murmurs.

23. _____ is the volume of blood pumped by the left ventricle into the aorta in one minute.
    a. Cardiac output
    b. Stroke volume
    c. Cardiac cycle
    d. Ventricular output

24. The volume of blood pumped by one ventricle during one beat is called the
    a. cardiac output.
    b. stroke volume.
    c. cardiac cycle.
    d. ventricular output.

25. Parasympathetic nerves release the neurotransmitter
    a. norepinephrine.
    b. epinephrine.
    c. acetylcholine.
    d. beta blockers.

26. Which of the following does not raise the heart rate?
    a. increased body temperature
    b. exercise
    c. stress
    d. decreased body temperature

Chapter

12

CIRCULATION OF BLOOD AND LYMPH

■ ■ ■

Outline

Introduction
I. Three main types of blood vessels are arteries, capillaries, and veins.
II. Blood circulates through two circuits.
   A. The pulmonary circulation carries blood to and from the lungs.
   B. The systemic circulation carries blood to the tissues.
      1. The aorta has four main regions.
      2. The superior and inferior venae cavae return blood to the heart.
      3. Four arteries supply the brain.
      4. The liver has an unusual circulation.
III. Several factors influence blood flow.
   A. The alternate expansion and recoil of an artery is its pulse.

B. Blood pressure depends on blood flow and resistance to blood flow.
   C. Pressure changes as blood flows through the systemic circulation.
   D. Blood pressure is expressed as systolic pressure over diastolic pressure.
   E. Blood pressure must be carefully regulated.
IV. The lymphatic system is a subsystem of the circulatory system.
   A. Lymph nodes filter lymph.
   B. Tonsils filter tissue fluid.
   C. The spleen filters blood.
   D. The thymus gland plays a role in immune function.

Learning Objectives

After you have studied this chapter, you should be able to:

1. Compare the structure and functions of arteries, capillaries, and veins.
2. Trace a drop of blood through the pulmonary and systemic circulations, listing the principal vessels and heart chambers through which it must pass on its journey from one part of the body to another. (For example, trace a drop of blood from the inferior vena cava to an organ such as the brain and then back to the heart.)
3. Identify the main divisions of the aorta and its principal branches.
4. Trace a drop of blood through the hepatic portal system.

5. Give the physiological basis for arterial pulse and describe how pulse is measured.
6. Describe the relationship of blood pressure to blood flow and resistance, and explain how blood pressure is measured.
7. Compare blood pressure in the different types of blood vessels of the systemic circulation.
8. Describe the mechanisms by which the nervous and endocrine systems regulate blood pressure.
9. Describe the tissues, organs, and functions of the lymphatic system.
10. Trace the flow of lymph from a lymph capillary to the left or right subclavian vein.

129

STUDY QUESTIONS

Within each category, fill in the blanks with the correct response.

INTRODUCTION

Blood vessels   Nourishes   Tissue fluid   Interstitial fluid   Smaller

1. _____ are the tubes that deliver blood to the tissues.

2. The _____ types of blood vessels are quite leaky.

3. When plasma enters the tissues it is called _____ or _____ fluid.

4. Interstitial fluid _____ the cells.

I. THREE MAIN TYPES OF BLOOD VESSELS ARE ARTERIES, CAPILLARIES, AND VEINS

Arteries   Connective   Macrophages   Veins   Arterioles   Metarterioles
Tunics   Capillaries   Exchanged   Oxygen   Valves   Collagen
Sinusoids   Venules   Heart   Pulmonary   Endothelium

1. _____ carry blood from the ventricles of the heart to each of the organs of the body.

2. All arteries except the _____ arteries carry blood rich in oxygen.

3. The smallest branches of an artery, called _____, are important in regulating blood pressure.

4. Blood flows from the arterioles through the _____.

5. Capillaries permit materials to be _____ between the blood and tissues.

6. Blood passes from the capillaries into _____ that conduct it back toward the heart.

7. The smallest veins are called _____.

8. All veins except the pulmonary vein carry blood that is poor in _____.

9. The wall of an artery or vein has three layers, or _____.

10. The inner layer of a blood vessel consists of _____ that forms a smooth surface for the blood.

11. The middle layer of a blood vessel consists of _____ tissue and smooth muscle.

12. The outer layer of a blood vessel consists of connective tissue that is rich in elastic and

_____ fibers.

13. Most large veins have _____ that permit the vein to conduct blood toward the

_____, even against the force of gravity.

14. The small vessels that directly link the arterioles with the venules are _____.

15. In the liver, spleen, and bone marrow, arterioles and venules are connected by capillarylike vessels called

_____.

16. _____ lie along the outer walls of sinusoids. They reach into the vessels to remove
worn-out blood cells and foreign matter from the circulation.

Labeling Exercise

Please fill in the correct labels for Figure 12-1.

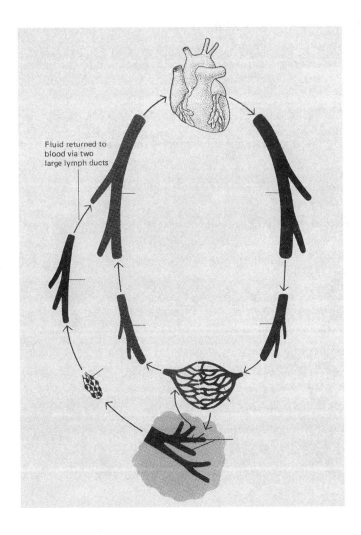

Fluid returned to
blood via two
large lymph ducts

Figure 12-1

II. BLOOD CIRCULATES THROUGH TWO CIRCUITS

Carbon dioxide Pulmonary Systemic Oxygen Right Ventricle

1. _____ circulation connects the heart with the lungs.

2. The _____ circulation connects the heart with all of the organs and tissues.

3. The left _____ pumps blood into the systemic circulation.

4. The _____ ventricle pumps blood into the pulmonary circulation.

5. As blood flows through the pulmonary capillaries, _____ diffuses out of the blood

   and _____ diffuses into it.

A. The Pulmonary Circulation Carries Blood To and From the Lungs

Atrium   Left atrium   Pulmonary   Pulmonary veins

1. Blood that is poor in oxygen returns from the systemic circulation to the right

   _____.

2. The _____ arteries deliver blood to the lungs.

3. The _____ return oxygen-rich blood to the _____.

4. Place numbers next to each item to indicate the correct sequence for pulmonary circulation.

   _____ Pulmonary arteries

   _____ Right ventricle

   _____ Right atrium

   _____ Pulmonary capillaries

   _____ Left atrium

   _____ Pulmonary veins

B. The Systemic Circulation Carries Blood to the Tissues

1. The Aorta Has Four Main Regions

Abdominal Ascending Thoracic Aortic arch Descending aorta

1. The _____ aorta is the first part of the aorta which travels upward (superiorly).

2. The _____ curves from the ascending aorta and makes a U-turn.

3. The _____ aorta descends from the aortic arch passing through the thorax. It lies posterior to the heart.

4. The _____ aorta is the region of the aorta below the diaphragm and is the longest region of the aorta.

5. The thoracic aorta and the abdominal aorta together make up the _____.

2. The Superior and Inferior Venae Cavae Return Blood to the Heart

Capillaries Inferior vena cava Superior vena cava Carbon dioxide Right atrium Veins

1. As blood circulates through the capillaries in the tissues, it delivers nutrients and oxygen to the cells and

   picks up _____.

2. _____ deliver blood to venules, which merge to form larger

   _____.

3. The _____ receives blood from the upper portions of the body.

4. The _____ receives blood returning from below the level of the diaphragm.

5. The superior and inferior venae cavae return blood to the _____ of the heart.

3. Four Arteries Supply the Brain

Anastomosis Brachiocephalic Internal carotid Venous sinuses Arteries
Circle of Willis Internal jugular Vertebral Basilar Heart Superior

1. Four _____ bring blood to the brain.

2. The two _____ arteries enter the cranial cavity in the midregion of the cranial floor.

3. The two _____ arteries pass through the foramen magnum and join on the ventral

   surface of the brain stem. Together, these arteries form the _____ artery.

4. The _____ is the circle of arteries at the base of the brain, formed by branches of the
   internal carotid arteries and the basilar artery.

5. _____ refers to the joining of two or more arteries.

6. From the brain capillaries, blood drains into large _____ located in the folds of the
   dura mater.

7. Blood from the venous sinuses empties into the _____ veins at either side of the
   neck.

8. From the internal jugular veins, blood passes through the _____ veins and into the

   _____ vena cava, which returns it to the _____.

9. Place numbers next to each item to indicate the correct sequence of blood flow to and from the brain.

   _____ Aorta

   _____ Superior vena cava

   _____ Common carotid artery

   _____ Circle of Willis

   _____ Internal carotid artery

   _____ Venous sinus

   _____ Capillaries in brain

   _____ Brachiocephalic vein

   _____ Internal jugular vein

Labeling Exercise

Please fill in the correct labels for Figure 12-2.

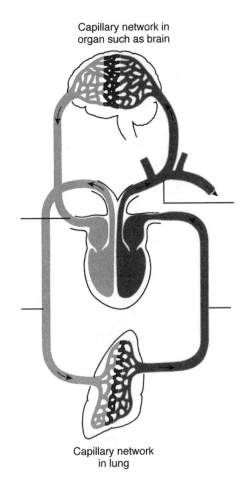

Capillary network in
organ such as brain

Capillary network
in lung

Figure 12-2

4.   *The Liver Has an Unusual Circulation*

Hepatic   Liver   Portal   Toxic   Homeostatic   Mesenteric   Superior mesenteric

1.   The body has a few specialized veins that carry blood to a second set of exchange vessels.   These veins are

     called _____ veins.

2.   The _____ portal vein delivers blood from the organs of the digestive system to the
     liver.

3.   Blood is delivered to the intestines by the _____ arteries.

4.   Blood, rich in nutrients, leaves the capillaries in the intestinal wall and flows into the

     _____ vein.

5. As blood flows through the sinusoids, _____ cells remove and store nutrients whose

   concentrations are above _____ levels.

6. Liver cells remove _____ substances from the blood.

III. SEVERAL FACTORS INFLUENCE BLOOD FLOW

A. The Alternate Expansion and Recoil of an Artery Is Its Pulse

Arterial   Diastole   Radial   Artery   Pulse   Systole   Carotid artery   Pumps blood

1. Each time the left ventricle _____ into the aorta, the elastic wall of the aorta stretches.

2. The alternate expansion and recoil of an artery is the _____ pulse.

3. As the left ventricle forces a large volume of blood into the aorta during _____, the aorta expands to accommodate it.

4. During _____, as the walls of the aorta recoil to normal size, the blood is kept flowing into the capillaries.

5. When you place your finger over an _____ near the skin surface, you can feel the pulse.

6. The _____ artery in the wrist is used most frequently to measure pulse. However,

   the common _____ in the neck region is often used as well.

7. Every time the heart contracts, a _____ wave is initiated.

B. Blood Pressure Depends on Blood Flow and Resistance to Blood Flow

Blood   **Diameter**   **Resistance**   **Blood pressure**   **Flow**
Viscosity   **Decreases**   **Volume**   **Peripheral resistance**

1. _____ is the force exerted by the blood against the inner walls of the blood vessels.

2. Blood pressure is determined by the _____ of blood and the

   _____ to the flow of blood.

3. When cardiac output increases, blood flow increases, causing a rise in _____ pressure.

4. The _____ of blood flowing through the body affects blood pressure.

5. Blood pressure _____ when blood volume is reduced.

6. _____ is the opposing force to blood flow caused by viscosity of the blood and by the friction between the blood and the wall of the blood vessel.

7. _____ remains fairly constant in a healthy person and is only a minor factor influencing changes in blood pressure.

8. A small change in _____ of a blood vessel causes a big change in blood pressure.

C.   Pressure Changes as Blood Flows Through the Systemic Circulation

Arterioles   **Blood flow**   **Heart**   **Veins**   **Baroreceptors**
Resistance   **Blood**   **Constrict**   **Valves**   **Blood pressure**

1. Because arteries are large, their walls do not present much _____ to blood flow.

2. _____ have a very small diameter and offer a great deal of resistance to blood flow.

3. _____ within the arteries is regulated mainly by the degree of constriction or dilation of the arterioles.

4. As blood flows through the capillaries, most of the pressure caused by the action of the

_____ is spent.

5. Veins offer little resistance to _____.

6. At any moment, more than half of all the blood in circulation can be found within the

_____.

7. Veins serve as a kind of _____ reservoir.

8. When blood is lost during hemorrhage, special receptors called _____ begin to

respond, causing the veins to _____.

9. _____ in the veins prevent backflow of blood that would otherwise occur because of the force of gravity.

D. Blood Pressure Is Expressed as Systolic Pressure Over Diastolic Pressure

Blood pressure	Diastolic	Normal	Stethoscope	Numerator	Sphygmomanometer
Hypertension	Diastole	Systole	Left ventricle	Denominator	Vascular resistance

1. In arteries, blood pressure rises during _____ and falls during

   _____ .

2. A _____ reading is expressed as systolic pressure over diastolic pressure.

3. _____ blood pressure for a young adult would be about 120/80.

4. In a blood pressure reading, systolic pressure is represented by the _____ and

   diastolic by the _____ .

5. Clinically, the most common way that blood pressure is measured is with a _____

   and _____ .

6. When the _____ pressure consistently measures more than 95 mm Hg, a person may

   be experiencing high blood pressure, or _____ .

7. In hypertension, there is usually increased _____ .

8. If high blood pressure persists, the _____ enlarges and may begin to deteriorate in
   function.

E. Blood Pressure Must Be Carefully Regulated

Aldosterone	Baroreceptors	Blood pressure	Renin	Blood volume
Angiotensin II	Angiotensinogen	Homeostatic	Vasodilation	Vasoconstriction

1. Blood pressure is kept within normal limits by the interaction of several complex

   _____ mechanisms.

2. When blood pressure falls, sympathetic nerves signal _____ in blood vessels so that
   pressure rises again.

3. When blood pressure increases, specialized receptors called _____ are affected.

4. Cardiac centers in the medulla inhibit sympathetic nerves that constrict arterioles; this action causes

   _____ , which lowers blood pressure.

5. In response to low blood pressure, the kidneys release the enzyme _____.

6. Renin acts on a plasma protein, _____, which initiates a series of reactions that

    produces _____, a hormone that acts as a powerful vasoconstrictor.

7. The hormone angiotensin II acts indirectly to maintain blood pressure by increasing the synthesis and release

    of the hormone _____ by the adrenal glands.

8. Aldosterone increases the retention of sodium ions by the kidneys, resulting in greater fluid retention and

    increased _____, which results in increased _____.

IV.   THE LYMPHATIC SYSTEM IS A SUBSYSTEM OF THE CIRCULATORY SYSTEM

Blood	**Lymph nodules**	**Lymphatics**	**Tissue (interstitial)**	**Drainage**
Lymphatic	**Lymphocytes**	**Lymph node**	**Lymphatic duct**	**Thoracic**

1. The _____ system is a subsystem of the circulatory system.

2. The lymphatic system consists of the clear, watery lymph that is formed from _____
    fluid.

3. The lymph tissue is a type of connective tissue with large numbers of _____.

4. The lymph system is organized into small masses of tissue called _____ and

    _____.

5. The lymph circulation is a(n) _____ system.

6. The job of the lymphatic system is to collect excess tissue fluid and return it to the

    _____.

7. Lymph capillaries conduct lymph to larger vessels called _____.

8. Lymphatic vessels from throughout the body except the upper right quadrant drain into the

    _____ duct.

9. Lymph from the lymphatic vessels in the upper right quadrant of the body drains into the right

    _____.

A. Lymph Nodes Filter Lymph

Axillary   Filter   Lymph nodes   Bacteria   Infection   Macrophages

1. _____ are masses of lymph tissue surrounded by a connective tissue capsule.

2. The main function of lymph nodes is to _____ the lymph.

3. Lymph nodes are most numerous in the _____ and groin regions, and many are located in the thorax and abdomen.

4. As lymph passes through lymph sinuses in lymph nodes, _____ and other phago-cytic cells remove bacteria and other foreign matter.

5. By filtering and destroying bacteria from the lymph, the lymph nodes help prevent the spread of

_____.

6. When _____ are present, lymph nodes may increase in size and become tender.

B. Tonsils Filter Tissue Fluid

Adenoids   Lingual   Pharyngeal   Tonsils   Filter   Palatine tonsils   Tonsillectomy

1. _____ are masses of lymph tissue located under the epithelial lining of the oral cavity and pharynx.

2. The major function of the tonsils is to _____ tissue fluid.

3. The _____ tonsils are located at the base of the tongue.

4. The _____ tonsil is located in the posterior wall of the nasal portion of the pharynx above the soft palate.

5. When enlarged, the pharyngeal tonsil is called the _____.

6. The _____ are oval masses of lymphatic tissue on each side of the throat.

7. The process of surgically removing the tonsils is called _____.

C.   The Spleen Filters Blood

Bacteria   Filter   Spleen   Splenectomy   Hemorrhage
Platelets   Blood   Liver   Macrophages   Bone marrow

1.   The _____ is the largest organ of the lymphatic system.

2.   Because it holds a great deal of _____, the spleen has a distinctive rich purple color.

3.   One of the main functions of the spleen is to _____ blood.

4.   As blood flows slowly through the spleen, _____ and other disease organisms are removed.

5.   _____ remove worn-out red and white blood cells and platelets in the spleen.

6.   A large percentage of the body's _____ are normally found in the spleen.

7.   When the spleen is ruptured, extensive—sometimes massive—_____ occurs.

8.   The procedure for surgically removing the spleen is called a _____.

9.   When the spleen is surgically removed, some of its functions are taken over by the

_____ and _____.

D.   The Thymus Gland Plays a Role in Immune Function

Hormones   Lymphocyte   Thymus gland   Immune   Puberty

1.   The _____ is a pinkish-gray lymphatic organ located in the upper thorax anterior to the great vessels as they emerge from the heart and posterior to the sternum.

2.   The thymus gland reaches its largest size at _____ and then begins to become smaller with age.

3.   The thymus gland plays a key role in the body's _____ processes.

4.   The thymus gland produces several _____ and also prepares one type of

_____ for action.

Labeling Exercise

Please fill in the correct labels for Figure 12-3.

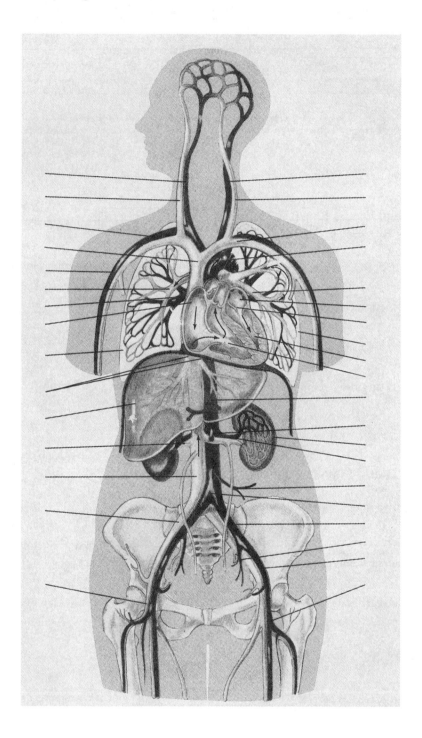

Figure 12-3

Labeling Exercise

Please fill in the correct labels for Figure 12-4.

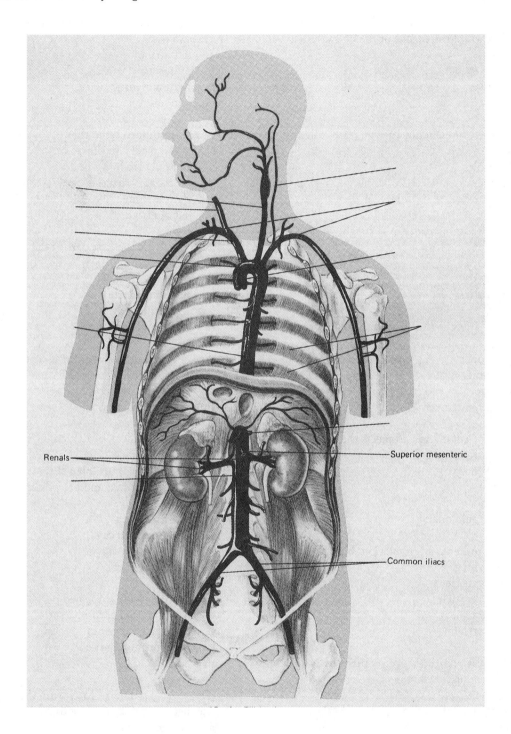

Renals

Superior mesenteric

Common iliacs

Figure 12-4

CHAPTER TEST

Select the correct response.

1. _____ carry blood from the ventricles of the heart to each of the organs of the body.
   a. Veins
   b. Arteries
   c. Venules
   d. Capillaries

2. The smallest branches of an artery are called
   a. veins.
   b. arterioles.
   c. venules.
   d. capillaries.

3. Blood flows from arterioles through
   a. arteries.
   b. veins.
   c. venules.
   d. capillaries.

4. The _____ circulation connects the heart with the lungs.
   a. pulmonary
   b. systemic
   c. cardiac
   d. cardiopulmonary

5. The _____ circulation connects the heart with all of the organs and tissues.
   a. pulmonary
   b. systemic
   c. cardiac
   d. cardiopulmonary

6. From the pulmonary circulation, blood is returned to the
   a. left ventricle.
   b. right ventricle.
   c. left atrium.
   d. right atrium.

7. Blood that is poor in oxygen returns from the systemic circulation to the
   a. left ventricle.
   b. right ventricle.
   c. left atrium.
   d. right atrium.

8. Blood is pumped into the right ventricle and then into the
   a. pulmonary veins.
   b. pulmonary arteries.
   c. right atrium.
   d. aorta.

9. Oxygen-rich blood returns from the pulmonary veins to the
   a. left atrium.
   b. pulmonary arteries.
   c. right atrium.
   d. left ventricle.

10. Blood is pumped from the _____ to the aorta, the largest artery in the body.
    a. right ventricle
    b. pulmonary arteries
    c. right atrium
    d. left ventricle

11. The _____ is the first part of the aorta, and it travels upward.
    a. thoracic aorta
    b. ascending aorta
    c. abdominal aorta
    d. aortic arch

12. The _____ curves from the ascending aorta and makes a U-turn.
    a. thoracic aorta
    b. superior vena cava
    c. abdominal aorta
    d. aortic arch

13. The _____ descends from the aortic arch, passes through the thorax, and lies posterior to the heart.
    a. thoracic aorta
    b. superior vena cava
    c. abdominal aorta
    d. ascending aorta

14. The basilar artery is formed by
    a. both internal carotid arteries.
    b. pulmonary arteries.
    c. both vertebral arteries.
    d. both a and c.

15. The _____ delivers blood from the organs of the digestive system to the liver.
    a. inferior vena cava
    b. superior vena cava
    c. hepatic portal vein
    d. pulmonary vein

16. Blood is delivered to the intestines by the
    a.   mesenteric veins.
    b.   mesenteric arteries.
    c.   superior vena cava.
    d.   carotid artery.

17. When cardiac output increases,
    a.   blood flow increases.
    b.   blood flow decreases.
    c.   blood pressure increases.
    d.   both a and c.

18. Blood can flow through the veins against gravity
    because
    a.   a system of valves prohibits backflow of
         blood.
    b.   most blood is found in the arteries, not in
         the veins.
    c.   veins are large and elastic and offer little
         resistance.
    d.   there is a lot of pressure in the veins keeping
         the blood moving at a rapid pace.

19. The principal function(s) of the lymphatic
    system is (are) to
    a.   collect and return tissue fluid to the blood.
    b.   defend the body against disease by producing
         lymphocytes.
    c.   absorb lipids from the intestine and trans-
         port them to the blood.
    d.   all of the above.

20. Which of the following is not part of the lymph
    system?
    a.   tonsils
    b.   lungs
    c.   thymus gland
    d.   spleen

21. Lymph is filtered by
    a.   lymphatics.
    b.   lymph nodes.
    c.   lungs.
    d.   liver.

22. The _____ is the largest organ of the lymphatic
    system.
    a.   spleen
    b.   liver
    c.   lymph node
    d.   lymphatics

Chapter

13

INTERNAL DEFENSE: IMMUNE RESPONSES

■ ■ ■

Outline

Introduction
I. Immune responses can be nonspecific or specific.
II. Nonspecific immune responses are rapid.
   A. Mechanical and chemical barriers prevent entry of most pathogens.
   B. Several types of proteins destroy pathogens.
      1. Cytokines are important signaling molecules.
      2. Complement leads to pathogen destruction.
   C. Phagocytes and natural killer cells destroy pathogens.
   D. Inflammation is a protective response.
III. Specific defense mechanisms include cell-mediated and antibody-mediated immunity.

A. Many types of cells participate in specific immune responses.
   1. Macrophages and dendritic cells present antigens.
   2. Lymphocytes are the principal warriors in specific immune responses.
B. T cells are responsible for cell-mediated immunity.
C. B cells are responsible for antibody-mediated immunity.
D. Long-term immunity depends on memory cells.
E. Active immunity can be induced by immunization.
F. Passive immunity is borrowed immunity.
IV. Immune responses are sometimes inadequate or harmful.

Learning Objectives

After you have studied this chapter, you should be able to:

1. Identify the body's ability to distinguish self from nonself as the basis for immune responses.
2. Contrast nonspecific and specific immune responses.
3. Describe several nonspecific immune responses including barriers, proteins such as cytokines and complement, phagocytosis, and inflammation.
4. Identify and give the functions of the principal cells of the immune system.
5. Describe cell-mediated immunity, including development of memory cells.

6. Describe antibody-mediated immunity, including the effects of antigen-antibody complex on pathogens both directly and through the complement system.
7. Compare primary and secondary immune responses.
8. Contrast active and passive immunity and give examples of each.
9. Describe several examples of immune malfunction.

STUDY QUESTIONS

Within each category, fill in the blanks with the correct response.

INTRODUCTION

Cell signaling   Immunology   Pathogens   Immune response   Messenger

1. Disease-causing organisms are referred to as _____.

2. _____ is the study of internal defense mechanisms.

3. A(n) _____ involves recognition of foreign molecules and a response aimed at eliminating them.

4. Immune responses depend on communication among cells, known as _____.

5. Cells of the immune system communicate directly with their surface molecules and indirectly by releasing

    _____ molecules.

I.   IMMUNE RESPONSES CAN BE NONSPECIFIC OR SPECIFIC

Antibodies   Nonspecific immune responses   Specific immune responses   Antigen   Pathogens

1. _____ provide general protection against pathogens.

2. Nonspecific immune responses prevent most _____ from entering the body.

3. _____ are precise responses against specific foreign molecules that have gained entrance to the body.

4. Any molecule that can be specifically recognized as foreign by cells of the immune system is called an

    _____.

5. An important specific defense mechanism is the production of _____.

II.   NONSPECIFIC IMMUNE RESPONSES ARE RAPID

Barriers   Inflammation   Proteins   Immune   Nonspecific

1. _____ defense mechanisms prevent pathogens from entering the body.

2. Nonspecific defense mechanisms include _____ that prevent pathogens from entering the body.

3. When pathogens succeed in penetrating the body, the _____ system responds quickly to destroy them.

4. Among the major nonspecific defenses are 1. _____ and cells that destroy pathogens,

and 2. _____ .

A.   Mechanical and Chemical Barriers Prevent Entry of Most Pathogens

Acids   Mucous   Respiratory   Bacteria   Nose   Skin   Enzymes   Pathogens   Sweat

1. Mechanical and chemical barriers prevent most _____ from entering the body.

2. The _____ and _____ membranes are the body's first line of defense against pathogens and other harmful substances.

3. The skin is populated by large numbers of harmless _____ that inhibit the multiplication of harmful bacteria that happen to land on it.

4. _____ and other secretions on the surface of the skin contain chemicals that destroy certain types of bacteria.

5. Pathogens that enter the body with inhaled air may be filtered out by hairs in the

_____ or trapped in the sticky mucous lining of the _____ passageway.

6. Bacteria that enter with food are usually destroyed by the _____ and

_____ of the stomach.

B.   Several Types of Proteins Destroy Pathogens

1.   *Cytokines Are Important Signaling Molecules*

Antiviral   Infecting   Interleukins   Machinery   Cytokines   Interferons   Lymphocytes

1. _____ are a large group of peptides and proteins that cells use to signal one another.

2. When infected by viruses or other intracellular parasites, cells respond by secreting cytokines called

_____ .

3. When viruses infect a cell, they take over the cellular _____ and use it to make more viruses.

4. Interferons signal neighboring cells and stimulate them to produce _____ proteins.

5. Viruses produced in cells exposed to interferon are less effective at _____ new cells.

6. _____ are a diverse group of proteins secreted mainly by macrophages and lymphocytes.

7. Interleukins regulate interaction between _____ and other cells of the body.

2. Complement Leads to Pathogen Destruction

Antigen   Complement   Pathogens   Cell wall   Destroy   Phagocytosis

1. _____ consists of more than 20 proteins present in plasma and other body fluids.

2. Normally, complement proteins are inactive until the body is exposed to a(n) _____.

3. Certain _____ activate the complement system directly.

4. Once activated, proteins of the complement system work to _____ pathogens.

5. Some complement proteins can rupture the _____ of the pathogen, while others

   promote _____ and inflammation.

C. Phagocytes and Natural Killer Cells Destroy Pathogens

Bacterium   Natural killer   Phagocytes   Target   Macrophages   Neutrophils   Phagocytosis

1. _____ are cells that ingest bacteria and other foreign matter.

2. In _____, a cell flows around a bacterium and engulfs it.

3. As a _____ is ingested, it is packaged within a vesicle formed by membrane pinched off from the plasma membrane.

4. _____ are the most common type of white blood cell.

5. Neutrophils and _____ are the phagocytes of the nonspecific immune system.

6. _____ cells are large, granular lymphocytes that originate in the bone marrow.

7. Natural killer cells destroy _____ cells by both nonspecific and specific antibody-requiring processes.

D.   Inflammation Is a Protective Response

Edema	Inflammation	Phagocytosis	Swelling	Fever	Interstitial	
Plasma	Heat	Mast	Redness	Histamine	Pain	Serotonin

1.   When pathogens invade tissues, _____ develops within a few hours.

2.   The clinical characteristics of inflammation are _____,

_____, _____, and _____.

3.   Inflammation is regulated by proteins in the _____, by cytokines, and by

_____ cells.

4.   Platelets, basophils, and mast cells release _____ and _____,
compounds that dilate blood vessels in the affected area and increase capillary permeability.

5.   Increased _____ seems to be one of the main functions of inflammation.

6.   As the volume of _____ fluid increases, edema, or _____,
occurs.

7.   _____ is a common clinical sign of widespread inflammatory response.

III.   SPECIFIC DEFENSE MECHANISMS INCLUDE CELL-MEDIATED AND ANTIBODY-MEDIATED IMMUNITY

Antibody-mediated   Cell-mediated   Lymphatic   Specific

1.   Several days are required to activate _____ immune responses.

2.   Specific immunity is the job of the _____ system.

3.   Two main types of specific immunity are _____ immunity and

_____ immunity.

A.   Many Types of Cells Participate in Specific Immune Responses

Dendritic   Lymphocytes   Macrophages   Neutrophils

1.   The principal warriors in specific immune responses are the _____.

2.   Other cell types that participate in specific immune responses are _____,

_____, and _____ cells.

1. Macrophages and Dendritic Cells Present Antigens

Digestive	Macrophages	Vaginal	Bacteria	Antigen-presenting
Interferons	Respiratory	Dendritic	Lysosomal	Urinary

1. Macrophages and _____ cells both develop from monocytes.

2. Macrophages secrete about 100 different compounds, including _____ and enzymes

   that destroy _____ .

3. When a macrophage ingests a bacterium, most, but not all, of the bacterial antigens are degraded by

   _____ enzymes.

4. Dendritic cells are strategically stationed in the skin and in the linings of the _____ ,

   _____ , _____ , and _____ passageways into the body.

5. Like _____ , dendritic cells capture foreign antigens and break them down.

6. Because they display fragments of foreign antigens as well as their own surface proteins, macrophage and

   dendritic cells are called _____ cells.

2. Lymphocytes Are the Principal Warriors in Specific Immune Responses

T	Cell-mediated	Natural killer	Thymus	Pathogens
B	Antibody-mediated	Bone marrow	Lymph	Plasma
Tumor	Immunological	Virally	Mutation	Stem cells

1. Three main types of lymphocytes are _____ lymphocytes,

   _____ lymphocytes, and _____ cells.

2. Natural killer cells kill _____ infected cells and _____ cells.

3. B cells are responsible for _____ immunity; they mature into

   _____ cells that produce specific antibodies.

4. T cells are responsible for _____ immunity.

5. T cells attack body cells infected by invading _____ , foreign cells, and cells altered

   by _____ .

6. B cells are produced in the _____ daily.

7. T cells and B cells originate from _____ in the bone marrow.

8. On their way to the _____ tissues, future T cells circulate through the

   _____ gland for processing.

9. The thymus gland makes T cells capable of _____ response.

B.   T Cells Are Responsible for Cell-Mediated Immunity

T   Cytotoxic T cells   Memory   Antigen   Enzymes   Mitosis   Cytokines   Helper   Suppress

1. In cell-mediated immunity, _____ cells attack invading pathogens directly.

2. There are thousands of different types of T cells, each capable of responding to a specific type of

   _____.

3. One group of T cells known as _____, or killer T cells, recognizes and destroys cells
   with foreign antigens on their surfaces.

4. Killer T cells kill their target cells by releasing a variety of _____ and

   _____ that destroy cells.

5. _____ T cells secrete cytokines that activate B cells and enhance immune responses.

6. Both helper T cells and cytotoxic T cells can _____ immune responses.

7. Once stimulated, T cells multiply by _____, each giving rise to a sizable clone of
   cells identical to itself.

8. Differentiated T cells remain in the lymph tissue as _____ T cells for years or even
   decades.

C.   B Cells Are Responsible for Antibody-Mediated Immunity

B	**Phagocytes**	**Antibodies**	**Plasma**	**Complement**
IgG	**Antigen**	**Deactivate**	**Receptor**	**Antigen-antibody**
Helper	**Pathogen**	**Memory**	**Lymph**	**Antigen-presenting**

1. _____ cells produce specific antibodies and send the antibodies out to perform their
   functions.

2. Only a B cell displaying a matching _____ on its surface can bind a particular

   _____.

3. In most cases, activation of B cells is a complex process that involves _____ cells and helper T cells.

4. _____ T cells secrete cytokines that help activate the B cells.

5. _____ cells are the mature B cells that secrete antibodies, which are carried by the

   _____ to the blood and are then transported to the infected region.

6. Some activated B cells become _____ B cells and continue for years to produce small amounts of antibody.

7. _____ are grouped into five classes according to their structure.

8. Normally, approximately 75% of the antibodies in the body belong in the _____ group.

9. The principal job of an antibody is to identify a _____ as foreign.

10. An antibody usually combines with several antigens, creating a mass of clumped

    _____ complex.

11. The antigen-antibody complex may _____ the pathogen or its toxin.

12. The antigen-antibody complex stimulates _____ to destroy the pathogen.

13. Antibodies of the IgG and IgM groups work by activating the _____ system.

D. Long-Term Immunity Depends on Memory Cells

T	Primary response	Antibodies	Memory
Killer	Immunity	Nonlymphatic	Secondary response

1. Memory B and memory T cells are responsible for long-term _____.

2. The first time we are exposed to an antigen, the body launches a _____.

3. Approximately 3 to 14 days are required to mobilize specific _____ cells and

   _____.

4. After an immune response, memory cells group strategically in many _____ tissues, including the lung, liver, kidney, and gut.

5. A second exposure to the same antigen, even years later, results in a _____, which is much more rapid than the primary response.

6. During a secondary response, memory T cells rapidly become _____ T cells that produce interferon and other substances that kill invading cells before we develop the disease.

7. It is because of _____ cells that we do not usually become ill from the same type of infection more than once.

E.   Active Immunity Can Be Induced by Immunization

Active immunity   Immunization   Vaccine   Antigens   Memory

1. _____ typically develops naturally from exposure to antigens and production of memory cells.

2. Active immunity can be artificially induced by _____; that is, by injection of a

_____.

3. Immunization causes your body to launch an immune response against the _____ in

the vaccine, which then results in the development of _____ cells.

F.   Passive Immunity Is Borrowed Immunity

Antibodies   Immunity   Passive   Effects   Memory   Pathogens   Immune response   Milk

1. In _____ immunity, an individual is given antibodies actively produced by other humans or animals.

2. Because passive immunity is borrowed immunity, its _____ do not last.

3. _____ produced by pregnant women cross the placenta and enter the blood of the fetus, giving the baby some protection for a few months after birth.

4. Babies who are breast-fed receive antibodies in their _____.

5. The antibodies that babies receive during breast-feeding provide _____ to the

pathogens responsible for gastrointestinal infection, and perhaps to other _____.

6. Passive immunity may only last for a few months because the body has not actively launched an

_____ and no _____ cells have been developed.

IV. IMMUNE RESPONSES ARE SOMETIMES INADEQUATE OR HARMFUL

Autoimmune	Immune	Antibodies	Helper	Immune function
Rejection	Cancer	Antigens	Acquired immunodeficiency syndrome	

1. Sometimes pathogens outmaneuver the _____ defenses and cause disease.

2. HIV, the virus that causes _____, infects _____ T cells.

3. Destruction of helper T cells seriously impairs _____ and puts the patient at risk for other infections.

4. Precancer cells have abnormal surface proteins that the immune system treats as foreign

   _____. Normally, the immune system responds to destroy them, but when the

   immune system is not effective, _____ develops.

5. During allergic reactions, the body produces _____ against mild antigens that normally do not stimulate an immune response.

6. In some cases, immune responses are directed against self, resulting in _____ diseases such as rheumatoid arthritis, multiple sclerosis, and insulin-dependent diabetes.

7. Transplanted tissues have foreign antigens that stimulate graft _____—an immune response in which T cells destroy the transplant.

CHAPTER TEST

Select the correct response.

1. _____ are organisms that cause disease.
   a. Pathogens
   b. Antigens
   c. Immunogens
   d. Antibodies

2. Which of the following ways can a disease-causing organism enter the body?
   a. wounds in the skin
   b. food
   c. copulation
   d. all of the above

3. Defense mechanisms depend on the body's ability to distinguish between itself and _____ that infect it.
   a. antigens
   b. antibodies
   c. pathogens
   d. lymphocytes

4. Any molecule that can be specifically recognized as foreign by cells of the immune system is called a(n)
   a. pathogen.
   b. antigen.
   c. immunoglobulin.
   d. antibody.

5. Nonspecific defense mechanisms include which of the following?
   a. skin
   b. T cells
   c. inflammation
   d. a and c

6. _____ is (are) a specific defense mechanism.
   a. Skin
   b. Mucus
   c. Stomach acids
   d. Lymphocytes

7. Specific defense is the function of the _____ system.
   a. circulatory
   b. endocrine
   c. lymphatic
   d. reproductive

8. A main type of lymphocyte is a
   a. T cell.
   b. lymph cell.
   c. B cell.
   d. a and c only.

9. In cell-mediated immunity, _____ cells attack invading pathogens directly.
   a. T
   b. B
   c. plasma
   d. red blood

10. T cells multiply by
    a. sexual reproduction.
    b. asexual reproduction.
    c. mitosis.
    d. osmosis.

11. _____ T cells combine with antigens on the surface of an invading cell.
    a. Memory
    b. Combination
    c. Killer
    d. Helper

12. _____ cells produce specific antibodies and send the antibodies out to perform their functions.
    a. T
    b. B
    c. Lymph
    d. Red blood

13. Which is not a type of T cell?
    a. memory
    b. killer
    c. helper
    d. antibody

14. Memory cells can develop from
    a. T cells.
    b. monocytes.
    c. B cells.
    d. both T and B cells.

15. _____ is not a class of antibodies.
    a. IgN
    b. IgG
    c. IgA
    d. IgM

16. Normally, approximately 75% of the antibodies in the body belong in the _____ group.
    a. IgG
    b. IgM
    c. IgA
    d. IgD

17. The principal function of an antibody is to identify a _____ as a foreign body.
    a. macrophage
    b. pathogen
    c. T cell
    d. B cell

18. Active immunity develops from exposure to
    a. lymph cells.
    b. antigens.
    c. antibodies.
    d. killer T cells.

19. Which of the following is not an autoimmune disease?
    a. multiple sclerosis
    b. rheumatoid arthritis
    c. insulin-dependent diabetes
    d. measles

CROSSWORD PUZZLE FOR CHAPTERS 10, 11, 12, AND 13

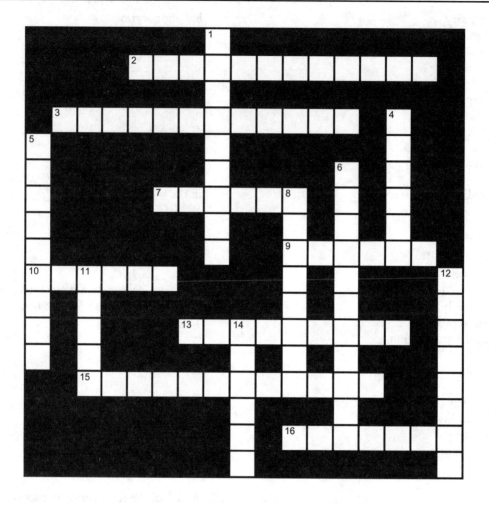

Across

2. Injection of a vaccine
3. Reaction to pathogen invasion
7. Serum plus clotting proteins
9. Function in cell-mediated immunity
10. Largest lymphatic organ
13. Cell fragments in the blood that function in clotting
15. High blood pressure
16. Period of contraction in the cardiac cycle

Down

1. The circulatory system that connects the heart and lungs
4. Artery in wrist commonly used to measure pulse
5. Atrioventricular valve on the right side of the heart
6. Proteins that trigger other cells to produce antiviral proteins
8. Proteins on red blood cell surfaces that determine blood type
11. Clear, watery fluid formed from tissue fluid
12. Vessels that carry blood away from the heart
14. Deficiency of red blood cells

Chapter

14

THE RESPIRATORY SYSTEM

■ ■ ■

Outline

Introduction
I. The respiratory system consists of the airway and lungs.
   A. The nasal cavities are lined with a mucous membrane.
   B. The pharynx is divided into three regions.
   C. The larynx contains the vocal cords.
   D. The trachea is supported by rings of cartilage.
   E. The bronchi enter the lungs.

F. Gas exchange occurs through the alveoli of the lungs.
G. The lungs provide a large surface area for gas exchange.
II. Ventilation moves air into and out of the lungs.
III. Gas exchange occurs by diffusion.
IV. Gases are transported by the circulatory system.
V. Respiration is regulated by the brain.
VI. The respiratory system defends itself against polluted air.

Learning Objectives

After you have studied this chapter, you should be able to:

1. Trace a breath of air through the respiratory system from nose to alveoli.
2. Describe the structure of the respiratory organs, including the lungs.
3. Compare and contrast inspiration and expiration.
4. Compare the process of oxygen and carbon dioxide exchange in the lungs with gas exchange in the tissues.

5. Compare the transport of oxygen and carbon dioxide in the blood.
6. Describe how the body regulates respiration.
7. Describe defense mechanisms that protect the lungs from pollutants in the air and describe some effects of breathing pollutants.

STUDY QUESTIONS

Within each category, fill in the blanks with the correct response.

INTRODUCTION

Carbon dioxide   Oxygen   Waste product   Cellular respiration   Respiration

1. _____ is the exchange of gases between the body and its environment.

2. Respiration supplies the cells of the body with _____ and rids them of

   _____.

3. _____ is the process by which cells capture energy from nutrients that serve as fuel molecules.

4. Oxygen is required for cellular respiration and carbon dioxide is produced as a

   _____.

I. THE RESPIRATORY SYSTEM CONSISTS OF THE AIRWAY AND LUNGS

Alveoli	Larynx	Bronchioles	Lung	Respiratory system
Bronchus	Oxygen	Trachea	Nostrils (nares)	

1. The _____ consists of the lungs and the airway.

2. A breath of air enters the body through the _____, the openings into the nose.

3. The _____ is also known as the voicebox.

4. The _____ is also known as the windpipe.

5. In order to enter the lungs, air must pass through the right or left _____.

6. From the bronchus, air passes into the many _____ of the lungs, which divide again

   and again until the air reaches the microscopic air sacs called _____.

7. _____ diffuses from the air sacs into the blood.

8. One bronchus enters each _____.

9. Trace the path that a breath of air would travel as it enters the body through the nose. Place a number next to each step in sequence starting with 1.

   _____ Pharynx

   _____ Nasal cavities

   _____ Trachea

   _____ Nostrils (nares)

   _____ Larynx

   _____ Alveoli

   _____ Bronchioles

   _____ Bronchus

A.   The Nasal Cavities Are Lined With a Mucous Membrane

Conchae	**Moistened**	**Nasal septum**	**Throat**	**Filtered**
Mucous	**Receptors**	**Hairs**	**Nares**	**Sinuses**

1. Air passes into the nose through its two openings, the nostrils, also called _____.

2. Coarse _____ in the nostrils prevent large particles from entering the nose.

3. The _____ is the partition that separates the nasal cavities.

4. The septum and walls of the nose consist of bone covered with a _____ membrane.

5. Three bony projections, the _____, project from the lateral walls of the nose.

6. As air passes through the nose, it is _____, _____, and brought to body temperature.

7. The nose also contains the _____ for the sense of smell.

8. Ciliated epithelial cells of the membrane push a steady stream of mucous, along with its trapped particles,

    toward the _____.

9. Several _____ in the bones of the skull communicate with the nasal cavities through small channels.

B.   The Pharynx Is Divided Into Three Regions

Esophagus   Larynx   Nasopharynx   Pharynx   Laryngopharynx   Mouth   Oropharynx

1. The nasal cavities are continuous with the _____.

2. Air enters the _____, the superior part of the pharynx.

3. From the nasopharynx, air moves down into the _____ behind the mouth.

4. The oropharynx receives food from the _____.

5. From the oropharynx, air passes through the _____ and enters the

    _____.

6. Behind the opening into the larynx, there is a second opening into the _____.

C. The Larynx Contains the Vocal Cords

Adam's apple   Glottis   Lungs   Cough   Laryngitis   Vocal cords   Epiglottis   Larynx

1. The _____, or voicebox, contains the vocal cords.

2. The opening into the larynx is called the _____.

3. The wall of the larynx is supported by cartilage that protrudes from the midline of the neck and is some

     times called the _____.

4. Inflammation of the larynx, or _____, is often caused by a respiratory infection or
     by irritating substances such as cigarette smoke.

5. The _____ are muscular folds of tissue that project from the lateral walls of the
     larynx.

6. The vocal cords vibrate as air from the _____ rushes past them during expiration.

7. During swallowing, a flap of tissue called the _____ automatically closes off the
     larynx so that food cannot enter the lower airway.

8. When the epiglottis fails to close properly, foreign matter comes into contact with the sensitive larynx,

     which causes a(n) _____ reflex.

D. The Trachea Is Supported by Rings of Cartilage

Cartilage   Lungs   Pharynx   Larynx   Mucous   Trachea

1. The _____, or windpipe, is located anterior to the esophagus.

2. The trachea extends from the _____ to the middle of the chest.

3. The trachea is kept from collapsing by rings of _____ in its wall.

4. The larynx, trachea, and bronchi are lined by a _____ membrane that traps dirt and
     foreign matter.

5. Ciliated cells in the mucous linings of the larynx, trachea, and bronchi continuously beat a stream of mucous

     upward to the _____, where it is swallowed.

6. The cilia-propelled mucus "elevator" keeps foreign material out of the _____.

E.   The Bronchi Enter the Lungs

Bronchial tree   Bronchi   Bronchioles   Lung

1.   The trachea divides into right and left _____.

2.   Each bronchus branches again and again, giving rise to smaller and smaller bronchi, and finally to very small

_____.

3.   The network of branching air passageways within the lungs is referred to as the

_____.

4.   There are more than 1 million bronchioles in each _____.

F.   Gas Exchange Occurs Through Alveoli of the Lungs

Alveoli   Breathing   Pulmonary surfactant   Alveolus   Capillaries

1.   Each bronchiole leads into a cluster of microscopic air sacs, the _____.

2.   The wall of a(n) _____ consists of a single layer of epithelial cells and elastic fibers

that permit it to stretch and contract during _____.

3.   Each alveolus is surrounded by a network of _____ so that gases diffuse easily
between the alveolus and blood.

4.   Alveoli are coated with a thin film of _____, a substance that prevents them from
collapsing.

G.   The Lungs Provide a Large Surface Area for Gas Exchange

Lungs	Pleural	Visceral	Hilus	Mediastinum
Lobes	Parietal	Thoracic	Diaphragm	Pleural cavity

1.   The _____ are large, paired organs that occupy the thoracic cavity.

2.   The lungs are separated medially by the _____.

3.   The right lung is divided into three _____.

4.   Each bronchus enters its lung at a depression called the _____.

5.   Each lung is covered with a _____ membrane, which forms a sac enclosing the lung,

and continues as the lining of the _____ cavity.

6. The part of the pleural membrane that covers the lung is the _____ pleura; the

portion that lines the thoracic cavity is the _____ pleura.

7. Between the pleural membranes is a potential space, the _____.

8. The floor of the thoracic cavity is a strong, dome-shaped muscle, the _____.

II. VENTILATION MOVES AIR INTO AND OUT OF THE LUNGS

Breathing   Diaphragm   Inspiration   Pulmonary   Collapsed lung   Expiration   Intercostal

1. _____ ventilation is the movement of air into and out of the lungs.

2. In general, we carry on pulmonary ventilation by _____.

3. The act of breathing in is called _____.

4. _____ is the process of breathing out.

5. During inspiration, the diaphragm contracts and flattens, and the _____ muscles contract.

6. Expiration occurs when the _____ and intercostal muscles relax.

7. A _____ occurs when the chest is punctured and the air sacs in the lungs collapse.

III. GAS EXCHANGE OCCURS BY DIFFUSION

Alveolus   Carbon dioxide   Diffuse   Oxygen   Breathing   Circulatory   Expired

1. _____ delivers oxygen to the alveoli of the lungs.

2. The vital link between the alveoli and the body cells is the _____ system.

3. Each _____ serves as a depot from which oxygen is loaded into the blood of the pulmonary capillaries.

4. The alveoli contain a greater concentration of _____ than the blood entering the pulmonary capillaries.

5. _____ moves from the blood, where it is more concentrated, to the alveoli, where it is less concentrated.

6. Oxygen and carbon dioxide _____ through the thin linings of the capillary and the alveolus.

7. _____ air contains 100 times more carbon dioxide than air from the environment.

IV.   GASES ARE TRANSPORTED BY THE CIRCULATORY SYSTEM

Bicarbonate ions   Hemoglobin   Oxygen   Plasma

1. When _____ diffuses into the blood, it enters the red blood cells and forms a weak chemical bond with hemoglobin, forming oxyhemoglobin.

2. Because the chemical bond linking oxygen with _____ is weak, this reaction is readily reversible.

3. Most of the carbon dioxide that is transported in the blood is transported as _____.

4. In the _____, carbon dioxide slowly combines with water to form carbonic acid.

V.   RESPIRATION IS REGULATED BY THE BRAIN

Blood   Cellular respiration   Respiratory failure   Cardiopulmonary resuscitation
Oxygen   Hyperventilate   Ventilation   Chemoreceptors
Breathing   Forcefully   Respiratory centers

1. Breathing is a rhythmic, involuntary process regulated by _____ in the brain stem.

2. Groups of neurons in the dorsal region of the medulla regulate the basic rhythm of

_____.

3. A group of neurons in the ventral region of the medulla becomes active only when we need to breathe

_____.

4. Overdose of certain medications such as barbiturates depresses the respiratory centers and may lead to

_____.

5. During exercise, the rate of _____ increases, producing more carbon dioxide; the

body must dispose of this carbon dioxide through increased _____.

6. Specialized _____ in the medulla and in the walls of the aorta and carotid arteries are sensitive to changes in arterial carbon dioxide concentration.

7. An increase in arterial carbon dioxide concentration results in a lowering of the pH of the

_____.

8. Surprisingly, _____ concentration generally does not play an important role in regulating respiration.

9. In order to stay under water longer, swimmers and divers voluntarily _____ before going under water in order to decrease the carbon dioxide content of the alveolar air and of the blood.

10. _____ is a method for aiding victims who have suffered respiratory and/or cardiac arrest.

VI. THE RESPIRATORY SYSTEM DEFENDS ITSELF AGAINST POLLUTED AIR

Bronchial Macrophages	Disease Carbon	Lymph Cilia	Respiratory Lung	Hair Mucous lining

1. The _____ system has a number of defense mechanisms that help protect the delicate lungs from damage.

2. The _____ in the nose and the _____ of the respiratory passageways help trap foreign particles in inspired air.

3. When we breathe dirty air, the _____ tubes narrow.

4. The smallest bronchioles and the alveoli are not equipped with mucus or cells with

   _____ .

5. Foreign particles that get through the respiratory defenses and find their way into the alveoli may remain

   there indefinitely, or they may be engulfed by _____ .

6. Macrophages may accumulate in the _____ tissue of the lungs.

7. Lung tissue of chronic smokers and those who work in dirty industrial environments contains large black

   ened areas where _____ particles have been deposited.

8. Continued insult to the respiratory system results in _____ .

9. Cigarette smoking is the main cause of _____ cancer.

Labeling Exercise

Please fill in the correct labels for Figure 14-1.

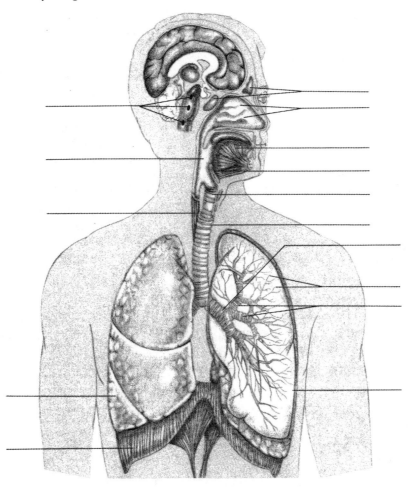

Figure 14-1

CHAPTER TEST

Select the correct response.

1. The process of respiration includes all of the following except
   a. breathing.
   b. gas exchange between the lungs and the blood.
   c. the formation of carbon deposits on the lungs.
   d. gas exchange between the blood and the cells.

2. The respiratory system consists of all of the following except
   a. lungs.
   b. esophagus.
   c. nose.
   d. trachea.

3. The correct order in which oxygen passes through the respiratory system is
   a. nasal cavities, larynx, pharynx, trachea, lungs.
   b. nasal cavities, trachea, larynx, pharynx, lungs.
   c. nasal cavities, pharynx, larynx, trachea, lungs.
   d. nasal cavities, pharynx, trachea, lungs, larynx.

4. Cells in the mucous lining of the nose
   a. produce about 1 half pint of mucus a day when there is a respiratory infection.
   b. trap dirt and particles that are inhaled through the nose.
   c. are swallowed with saliva.
   d. all of the above.

5. The pharynx consists of the
   a. nasopharynx.
   b. oropharynx.
   c. laryngopharynx.
   d. all of the above.

6. The inside of the lungs consists of all of the following except
   a. bronchi.
   b. bronchioles.
   c. alveoli.
   d. villi.

7. The surface area of the lungs through which gases can be exchanged is about the size of
   a. 1 square meter.
   b. a tennis court.
   c. a soccer field.
   d. a football field.

8. During expiration, _____ does not occur.
   a. diaphragm and intercostal muscle contraction
   b. decrease of volume of thoracic cavity
   c. lung recoil
   d. decrease of lung volume

9. Carbon dioxide is transported in the blood
   a. as a compound called bicarbonate.
   b. attached to hemoglobin.
   c. by dissolving in the plasma.
   d. all of the above.

10. The normal adult breathing rate is approximately _____ breaths per minute.
    a. 1 to 10
    b. 12 to 20
    c. 20 to 28
    d. 28 to 35

11. Respiratory centers in the pons and the medulla regulate the
    a. rate of breathing.
    b. depth of breathing.
    c. rhythm of breathing.
    d. all of the above.

12. Cardiopulmonary resuscitation (CPR) must be started immediately because brain damage may occur within _____ minutes of respiratory arrest.
    a. 4
    b. 12
    c. 20
    d. 60

13. Which of the following are pulmonary diseases that have been linked to smoking and breathing dirty air?
    a. emphysema
    b. chronic bronchitis
    c. lung cancer
    d. all of the above

Chapter

15

THE DIGESTIVE SYSTEM

■ ■ ■

Outline

Introduction
I. The digestive system processes food.
II. The digestive system consists of the digestive tract and accessory organs.
   A. The wall of the digestive tract has four layers.
   B. Folds of the peritoneum support the digestive organs.
   C. The mouth ingests food.
      1. The teeth break down food.
      2. The salivary glands produce saliva.
   D. The pharynx is important in swallowing.
   E. The esophagus conducts food to the stomach.
   F. The stomach digests food.

   G. Most digestion takes place in the small intestine.
   H. The pancreas secretes enzymes.
   I. The liver secretes bile.
III. Digestion occurs as food moves through the digestive tract.
   A. Glucose is the main product of carbohydrate digestion.
   B. Bile emulsifies fat.
   C. Proteins are digested to free amino acids.
IV. The intestinal villi absorb nutrients.
V. The large intestine eliminates wastes.
VI. A balanced diet is necessary to maintain health.
VII. Energy metabolism is balanced when energy input equals energy output.

Learning Objectives

After you have studied this chapter, you should be able to:

1. Describe in general terms the following steps in processing food: ingestion, digestion, absorption, and elimination.
2. List in sequence each structure through which a bite of food passes on its way through the digestive tract; label a diagram of the digestive system.
3. Describe the wall of the digestive tract, distinguish between the visceral peritoneum and the parietal peritoneum, and describe their major folds.
4. Describe the structures of the mouth, including the teeth, and give their functions.
5. Describe the structure and function of the pharynx and esophagus.
6. Describe the structure of the stomach and its role in processing food.

7. Identify the three main regions of the small intestine and give the function of the small intestine.
8. Summarize the functions of the pancreas and liver.
9. Summarize carbohydrate, lipid, and protein digestion.
10. Describe the structure of an intestinal villus and explain the role of villi in absorption of nutrients.
11. Describe the structure and functions of the large intestine.
12. List the nutrients that make up a balanced diet and summarize the functions of each.
13. Contrast basal metabolic rate with total metabolic rate, and write the basic energy equation for maintaining body weight.

STUDY QUESTIONS

Within each category, fill in the blanks with the correct response.

INTRODUCTION

Digestive   Energy   Nutrients   Nutrition

1. _____ are the substances in food that are used as building blocks to make new cells and tissues.

2. Some nutrients serve as a(n) _____ source to run the machinery of the body.

3. The process of taking in and using food is _____ .

4. The _____ system processes the food and breaks it down into a form that can be delivered to the cells and then used by the cells.

I. THE DIGESTIVE SYSTEM PROCESSES FOOD

Absorption   Digestion   Ingestion   Mechanical   Chemical   Elimination   Liver

1. _____ involves taking food into the mouth, chewing it, and then swallowing it.

2. _____ is the breakdown of food into smaller molecules.

3. _____ digestion is the process of breaking down pieces of food by chewing and by churning and mixing movements in the stomach.

4. _____ digestion is the process of breaking down large molecules including carbohydrates, proteins, and fats into small molecules that can be absorbed from the digestive tract and used by the cells of the body.

5. _____ is the transfer of digested food through the wall of the intestine and into the circulatory system.

6. _____ removes undigested and unabsorbed food from the body.

7. The circulatory system transports the food molecules, or nutrients, to the _____ , where many are removed and stored.

II. THE DIGESTIVE SYSTEM CONSISTS OF THE DIGESTIVE TRACT AND ACCESSORY ORGANS

Alimentary   Gastrointestinal   Mouth   Salivary   Anus   Liver   Pancreas

1. The digestive tract, also called the _____ canal, is a tube approximately 4.4 m long.

2. The digestive tract extends from the _____, where food is taken in, to the

    _____, through which unused food is eliminated.

3. Below the diaphragm, the digestive tract is often referred to as the _____ tract.

4. Three types of accessory digestive glands are the _____ glands,

    _____, and _____. These are not part of the digestive tract,
    but they secrete digestive juices into it.

5. Place the correct number next to each choice to indicate the proper sequence.

    _____ Esophagus

    _____ Mouth

    _____ Stomach

    _____ Pharynx

    _____ Large intestine

    _____ Small intestine

A. The Wall of the Digestive Tract Has Four Layers

Connective	**Epithelial**	**Submucosa**	**Digestion**	**Parietal peritoneum**
Peristalsis	**Digestive**	**Peritonitis**	**Mucosa**	**Peritoneal cavity**

1. From the esophagus to the anus, the wall of the _____ tract consists of four layers.

2. The _____ is the lining of the digestive tract. It consists of

    _____ tissue resting on a layer of loose connective tissue.

3. In the stomach and small intestine, the mucosa is thrown into folds, which greatly increase its surface area

    for _____ and absorption.

4. Beneath the mucosa lies a layer of connective tissue called the _____ which is rich in
    blood vessels and nerves.

5. The third layer of the digestive system consists of muscle. This muscle contracts in a wavelike motion called

    _____, which pushes food through the digestive tract.

6. The outer coating of the wall of the digestive tract consists of _____ tissue.

7. The _____ is the sheet of connective tissue that lines the walls of the abdominal and pelvic cavities.

8. Between the visceral and parietal peritoneum is a potential space called the _____.

9. Inflammation of the peritoneum, called _____, can have very serious consequences, because infection can easily spread to adjoining organs.

B.   FOLDS OF THE PERITONEUM SUPPORT THE DIGESTIVE ORGANS

Greater omentum   Lesser omentum   Mesocolon   Intestine   Mesentery   Peritoneum

1. The _____, a large double fold of peritoneal tissue, extends from the parietal peritoneum and attaches to the small intestine.

2. The mesentery anchors the _____ to the posterior abdominal wall.

3. Other important folds of the _____ are the greater omentum, the lesser omentum, and the mesocolon.

4. The _____, also known as the "fatty apron," is a large double fold of peritoneum attached to the stomach and intestine.

5. The _____ suspends the stomach and duodenum from the liver.

6. The _____ is a fold of peritoneum that attaches the colon to the posterior abdominal wall.

C.   The Mouth Ingests Food

Mechanical   Oral cavity   Taste buds   Tongue

1. The mouth, or _____, ingests food and begins the process of digestion.

2. _____ digestion begins as you bite, grind, and chew food with your teeth.

3. The flexible, muscular _____ on the floor of the mouth pushes the food around, which aids in chewing and swallowing.

4. _____ on the tongue enable us to taste foods as sweet, sour, salty, or bitter.

1.   The Teeth Break Down Food

Alveolar	**Deciduous**	**Roots**	**Dentin**	**Pulp**	**Root canals**
Canines	**Crown**	**Incisor**	**Enamel**	**Pulp cavity**	

1. The teeth are rooted in sockets of the _____ processes.

2. Each tooth consists of a(n) _____, the portion above the gum, and one or more

    _____, the portion beneath the gum line.

3. Teeth are composed mainly of _____, a calcified connective tissue that imparts shape
    and rigidity to the tooth.

4. In the crown region of the tooth, the dentin is protected by a tough covering of

    _____.

5. The dentin encloses a _____ filled with _____, an extremely
    sensitive connective tissue containing blood vessels and nerves.

6. Narrow extensions of the pulp cavity, called _____, pass through the roots of the
    tooth.

7. Baby teeth, or _____ teeth, start showing their crowns above the gums by about 6
    months of age.

8. The _____ teeth are specialized for biting and cutting.

9. Lateral to the incisors are the _____, which assist humans in biting, but are enlarged
    in many mammals and are adapted for stabbing and tearing prey.

Labeling Exercise

Please fill in the correct labels for Figure 15-1.

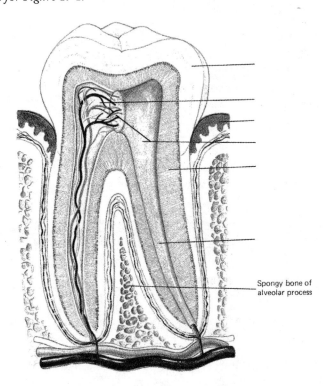

Spongy bone of
alveolar process

Figure 15-1

2. The Salivary Glands Produce Saliva

Bolus   Saliva   Sublingual   Parotid   Salivary amylase   Submandibular

1. The _____ glands are the largest salivary glands.

2. The _____ glands lie below the jaw.

3. The _____ glands are under the tongue.

4. _____ consists of two main components: (1) a thin, watery secretion containing

   _____, a digestive enzyme, and (2) a mucous secretion that lubricates the mouth.

5. By moistening food, saliva helps the tongue convert a mouthful of food to a semisolid mass called a(n)

   _____.

D.   The Pharynx Is Important in Swallowing

Epiglottis   Swallowing   Oropharynx   Esophagus   Tongue   Nasopharynx
Pharynx   Laryngopharynx   Uvula   Soft palate Hard palate

1. _____ moves the bolus from the mouth through the pharynx and down the esophagus.

2. The _____, or throat, is a muscular tube approximately 12 cm long that serves as the
   hallway for both the respiratory and digestive systems.

3. The three regions of the pharynx are the _____, posterior to the mouth; the

   _____, posterior to the nose; and the _____, which opens
   into the larynx and esophagus.

4. The oropharynx and the nasopharynx are partitioned by the _____.

5. The muscular soft palate is a posterior extension of the bony _____, which serves as
   the roof of the mouth.

6. A small mass of tissue, the _____, hangs from the lower border of the soft palate.

7. During swallowing, the bolus is forced into the oropharynx by the _____.

8. Reflex contractions of muscles in the wall of the pharynx propel the food into the

   _____.

9. During swallowing, the opening to the larynx is closed by a small flap of tissue called the

    _____.

E.   The Esophagus Conducts Food to the Stomach

Esophagus   Peristaltic   Sphincter   Heartburn   Pharynx   Stomach

1. The esophagus extends from the _____ through the thoracic cavity.

2. The esophagus passes through the diaphragm and empties into the _____.

3. The bolus is swept through the pharynx and into the esophagus by _____ waves of muscle contraction.

4. At the lower end of the esophagus is a circular muscle called a(n) _____ muscle.

5. The sphincter muscle prevents the highly acidic gastric juices from splashing up into the

    _____.

6. Occasionally, gastric juice spurts up into the esophagus, the wall of the esophagus becomes irritated, and the

    resulting spasms cause _____.

F.   The Stomach Digests Food

Cardiac   Glands   Peristalsis   Small intestine   Chyme   Mucus
Pyloric   Stomach   Contractions   Pepsinogen   Rugae

1. When a peristaltic wave passes down the esophagus, the _____ sphincter relaxes,

    permitting the bolus to enter the _____.

2. When empty, the lining of the stomach has many folds, which are called _____.

3. _____ of the stomach mix the food thoroughly.

4. The stomach mashes and churns food and moves it along by _____.

5. The stomach is lined with simple epithelium that secretes large amounts of _____.

6. Millions of gastric _____ in the wall of the stomach secrete hydrochloric acid and enzymes.

7. Chief cells in the gastric glands secrete _____, an inactive form of the enzyme pepsin, which begins the digestion of proteins.

8. As food is digested over a period of 3 to 4 hours, it is converted into a soupy mixture called

    _____.

9. The exit of the stomach is guarded by the _____ sphincter, a strong ring of muscle.

10. When the pyloric sphincter relaxes, chyme passes into the _____.

G.   Most Digestion Takes Place in the Small Intestine

Absorption	**Goblet cells**	**Jejunum**	**Ileum**	**Intestinal glands**
Duodenum	**Digestion**	**Pancreas**	**Villi**	**Small intestine**

1. The _____ is a coiled tube more than 5 m long and 4 cm in diameter.

2. The first 22 cm or so of the small intestine make up the _____, which is curved like the letter C.

3. The portion of the small intestine that curves downward is called the _____, and it extends for approximately 2 m; the last portion of the small intestine is called the

    _____.

4. The lining of the small intestine has millions of tiny fingerlike projections called

    _____.

5. The villi increase the surface area of the small intestine so that there is greater surface area for digestion and

    _____ of nutrients.

6. Most _____ takes place in the duodenum rather than in the stomach.

7. _____ secrete large amounts of fluid that help keep the chyme in a fluid state so that nutrients can be easily absorbed.

8. _____ in the mucosa secrete alkaline mucus that helps protect the intestinal wall from the acidic chyme and from the action of digestive enzymes.

9. The liver and _____ release digestive juices into the duodenum that act on the chyme.

H.   The Pancreas Secretes Enzymes

Acute pancreatitis   Enzymes   Pancreas   Duodenum   Exocrine   Pancreatic

1.   The _____ is a long, large gland that lies in the abdomen inferior to the stomach.

2.   The pancreas is both an endocrine and a(n) _____ gland.

3.   The exocrine portion of the pancreas secretes _____ juice, which contains a number

of _____ .

4.   The pancreatic duct from the pancreas joins the duct coming from the liver, forming a single duct that passes

into the _____ .

5.   If the pancreatic ducts are blocked, the pancreas may be digested by its own enzymes. This condition is

called _____ , and is frequently associated with alcoholism.

I.   The Liver Secretes Bile

Bile   Hepatic   Liver cell   Common bile duct   Intestine   Lobe   Gallbladder   Liver   Portal

1.   The _____ is the largest and one of the most complex organs in the body.

2.   A single _____ can carry on more than 500 separate metabolic activities.

3.   The right _____ of the liver is larger than its left one and has three main parts.

4.   Oxygen-rich blood is brought to the liver by the _____ arteries.

5.   The liver also receives blood from the hepatic _____ vein.

6.   The hepatic portal vein delivers nutrients absorbed from the _____ .

7.   The liver produces and secretes _____ , which is important in the mechanical digestion of fats.

8.   Bile is stored in the pear-shaped _____ .

9.   The cystic duct from the gallbladder joins the hepatic duct from the liver to form the

_____ , which opens into the duodenum.

III. DIGESTION OCCURS AS FOOD MOVES THROUGH THE DIGESTIVE TRACT

Chyme   Gastrin   Reflexes

1. Secretion of digestive juices is stimulated by hormones and _____.

2. The hormone _____, which is released by the stomach mucosa, stimulates the gastric glands to secrete.

3. The intestinal glands are stimulated to release their fluid mainly by local _____ that occur when the small intestine is stretched by chyme.

A. Glucose Is the Main Product of Carbohydrate Digestion

Maltase   Glucose   Maltose   Pancreatic amylase   Carbohydrate
Lactose   Mouth   Sucrose   Salivary amylase

1. Large carbohydrates such as starch and glycogen consist of long chains of _____ molecules.

2. Starch digestion begins in the _____.

3. In the mouth, the enzyme _____ begins breaking down some of the long starch

    molecules to smaller compounds and then to the sugar _____.

4. In the duodenum, _____, an enzyme in the pancreatic juice, splits remaining starch molecules to maltose.

5. The enzyme _____ breaks down each maltose molecule to two molecules of glucose.

6. _____, the sugar we use in our coffee, and _____, milk sugar, are also broken down to simple sugars in the duodenum.

7. Glucose is the major product of _____ digestion.

B. Bile Emulsifies Fat

Bile   Fatty acids   Lipase   Duodenum   Glycerol   Triglycerides

1. Digestion of fat takes place mainly in the _____.

2. _____ emulsifies fat by a detergent action that breaks down large fat droplets into smaller droplets.

3. Small fat droplets are acted on by an enzyme in the pancreatic juice called _____.

4. Pancreatic lipase breaks down _____ to free _____ and

_____ .

C.   Proteins Are Digested to Free Amino Acids

Amino acids   Pepsin   Protein   Trypsin   Peptide   Polypeptides   Stomach

1. Proteins consist of smaller molecules called _____ .

2. Amino acid subunits are linked together by chemical bonds called _____ bonds.

3. The goal of _____ digestion are free amino acids.

4. Protein digestion begins in the _____ , with the enzyme

_____ .

5. Pepsin breaks down most proteins to smaller molecules called _____ .

6. In the duodenum, the enzyme _____ in the pancreatic juice breaks down proteins
    and polypeptides.

IV.   THE INTESTINAL VILLI ABSORB NUTRIENTS

Absorbed   Lacteal   Villi   Fatty acids   Liver   Villus

1. After food has been digested, the nutrients are absorbed by the intestinal _____ .

2. Within each _____ is a network of capillaries that branch from an arteriole and
    empty into a venule.

3. A central lymph vessel called a _____ is also present inside the villus.

4. Amino acids and simple sugars are _____ into the blood.

5. Amino acids and simple sugars are transported directly to the _____ by the hepatic
    portal vein.

6. _____ are absorbed into the lacteals.

V. THE LARGE INTESTINE ELIMINATES WASTES

Anal canal	**Feces**	**Peristaltic**	**Appendicitis**	**Vermiform appendix**
Defecate	**Rectum**	**Cecum**	**Transverse colon**	**Ascending colon**
Chyme	**Colon**	**Ileocecal**	**Sigmoid colon**	

1. After the _____ has passed through the stomach and small intestine, it consists mainly of water and indigestible wastes such as cellulose.

2. The small intestine is separated from the large intestine by the _____ valve.

3. When a _____ contraction brings chyme toward it, the ileocecal valve opens, allowing the chyme to enter the large intestine.

4. The first 7 cm of the large intestine is a pouch called the _____.

5. The _____, a worm-shaped blind tube, hangs down from the end of the cecum.

6. Inflammation of the appendix, called _____, can lead to peritonitis and other complications if not diagnosed and treated promptly.

7. From the cecum to the rectum, the large intestine is called the _____.

8. The _____ extends from the cecum straight up to the lower border of the liver.

9. As the ascending colon turns horizontally, it becomes the _____.

10. On the left side of the abdomen, the descending colon turns downward and forms the S-shaped

    _____, which empties into the short _____.

11. The last 4 cm of the rectum are called the _____.

12. As chyme slowly passes through the large intestine, water and sodium are absorbed from it; what remains

    becomes _____.

13. After meals, contractions of the large intestine increase. This stimulates the desire to

    _____.

VI. A BALANCED DIET IS NECESSARY TO MAINTAIN HEALTH

Antioxidants	**Oxidants**	**Water**	**Carbohydrates**	**Essential amino acids**
Lipids	**Proteins**	**Minerals**	**Energy sources**	**Vitamins**

1. Carbohydrates, lipids, and proteins can all be used as _____.

2. _____ is one of the main components of the body and is used by the body to transport materials.

3. _____ are inorganic nutrients ingested in the form of salts dissolved in food and water.

4. _____ are organic compounds required for certain reactions to take place. Many of these serve as coenzymes, compounds that work with enzymes to regulate chemical reactions.

5. _____ are ingested mainly as starch or cellulose. These are digested to glucose or other simple sugars, which can be absorbed into the blood.

6. Most of the _____ we ingest are fats or cholesterols.

7. _____ are digested into their component amino acids. Proteins are the essential building blocks of cells, and many serve as enzymes.

8. Of the 20 or so amino acids, nine are considered _____ because they must be provided in the diet.

9. _____ are highly reactive molecules that can damage DNA and other cell molecules by snatching electrons.

10. Some phytochemicals are _____ that destroy oxidants.

VII.   ENERGY METABOLISM IS BALANCED WHEN ENERGY INPUT EQUALS ENERGY OUTPUT

Malnutrition	**Stored fat**	**Decreases**	**Basal metabolic rate**
Metabolic rate	**Heat**	**Obesity**	**Total metabolic rate**

1. The amount of energy released by the body per unit of time is a measure of _____.

2. Much of the energy expended by the body is ultimately converted to _____.

3. The _____ is the rate at which the body releases heat as a result of breaking down fuel molecules.

4. An individual's _____ is the sum of the basal metabolic rate and the energy used to carry on all daily activities.

5. When energy output is greater than energy input, _____ is burned and body weight

    _____.

6. _____, or poor nutritional status, can result from dietary intake that is either above or below required needs.

7. _____ is a serious nutritional problem in which energy imbalance results in the deposit of an excess amount of fat in adipose tissues.

Labeling Exercise

Please fill in the correct labels for Figure 15-2.

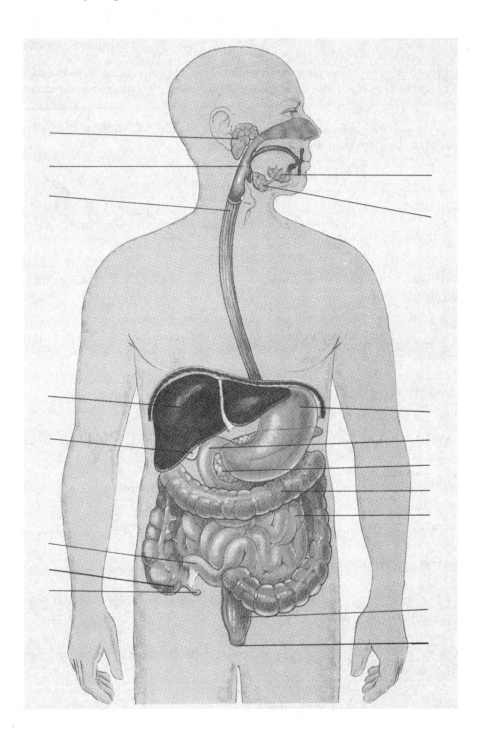

Figure 15-2

CHAPTER TEST

Select the correct response.

1. The sequence of the parts of the digestive tract through which food passes is
   a. mouth, esophagus, pharynx, stomach, small intestine, and large intestine.
   b. mouth, pharynx, esophagus, stomach, small intestine, and large intestine.
   c. mouth, esophagus, stomach, pharynx, small intestine, and large intestine.
   d. mouth, pharynx, esophagus, stomach, large intestine, and small intestine.

2. The sequence of the four major processes of the digestive system is
   a. digestion, absorption, ingestion, and elimination.
   b. digestion, indigestion, absorption, and elimination.
   c. ingestion, indigestion, digestion, and elimination.
   d. ingestion, digestion, absorption, and elimination.

3. Important folds of the peritoneum include the
   a. mesentery.
   b. greater omentum.
   c. lesser omentum.
   d. all of the above.

4. Taste buds on the tongue enable us to taste
   a. sweet.
   b. sour.
   c. salty.
   d. all of the above.

5. The three main pairs of salivary glands are
   a. parotid, submandibular, and sublingual.
   b. parotid, inframandibular, and bilingual.
   c. submandibular, supramandibular, and sublingual.
   d. submandibular, sublingual, and bilingual.

6. The three regions of the pharynx are
   a. oropharynx, esophagopharynx, and nasopharynx.
   b. oropharynx, nasopharynx, and hepatopharynx.
   c. oropharynx, nasopharynx, and laryngopharynx.
   d. laryngopharynx, nasopharynx, and esophagopharynx.

7. If the lining of the small intestine could be completely unfolded and spread out, its surface would approximate the size of a
   a. football field.
   b. tennis court.
   c. basketball court.
   d. racquetball court.

8. Most digestion takes place in the
   a. small intestine.
   b. stomach.
   c. large intestine.
   d. esophagus.

9. Which of the following is not a function of the liver?
   a. secretes bile
   b. removes nutrients from blood
   c. converts glucose to glycogen
   d. digests carbohydrates

10. Starch digestion begins in the
    a. mouth.
    b. esophagus.
    c. stomach.
    d. small intestine.

11. Fat digestion takes place mainly in the
    a. mouth.
    b. esophagus.
    c. stomach.
    d. duodenum.

12. Protein digestion begins in the
    a. mouth.
    b. esophagus.
    c. stomach.
    d. small intestine.

13. The function of the vermiform appendix is
    a. to store bile.
    b. to store fats.
    c. to store certain vitamins.
    d. unknown.

14. _____ is not a function of the large intestine.
    a. Absorption
    b. Incubation of bacteria
    c. Digestion
    d. Elimination of wastes

15. Nutrients required for good health are provided in a balanced diet and consist of all but which of the following?
   a. water
   b. lipids
   c. vitamins
   d. alcohol

16. Sugars account for 25% of the _____ we ingest.
   a. proteins
   b. carbohydrates
   c. fats
   d. minerals

17. In order for a person to lose weight, which of the following must happen?
   a. Calories taken in must be greater than calories expended.
   b. Calories taken in must be less than calories expended.
   c. Calories taken in must be exactly equal to calories expended.
   d. Calories play very little role in weight loss.

CROSSWORD PUZZLE FOR CHAPTERS 14 AND 15

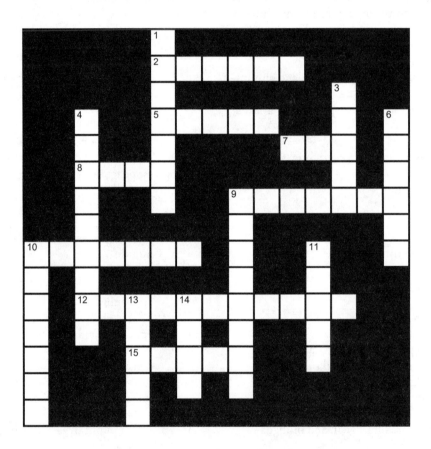

Across
2. Contains vocal cords
5. Large intestine from cecum to rectum
7. Number of bronchi
8. Opening for elimination of feces
9. Windpipe
10. Large salivary gland
12. Stores bile
15. Absorb nutrients

Down
1. During digestion, many carbohydrates are broken down into these components
3. Consists of crown and roots
4. Large muscle that functions in breathing
6. Digests fat
9. Cavity in which lungs are located
10. Throat
11. Terminal part of small intestine
13. Large organ that lies inferior to diaphragm
14. Produced by liver

Chapter

16

THE URINARY SYSTEM
AND FLUID BALANCE

■ ■ ■

Outline

Introduction

I. Metabolic waste products include water, carbon dioxide, and nitrogenous wastes.

II. The urinary system has many regulatory functions.

III. The urinary system consists of the kidneys, urinary bladder, and their ducts.
   A. The kidneys consist of a cortex and medulla.
   B. The nephrons are the functional units of the kidney.
   C. Urine is transported by ducts and stored in the bladder.
   D. Urination empties the bladder.

IV. Urine is produced by filtration, reabsorption, and secretion.
   A. Glomerular filtration is not selective with regard to small molecules and ions.

B. Tubular reabsorption is highly selective.

C. Some substances are secreted from the blood into the filtrate.

D. Urine consists mainly of water.

V. Urine volume and composition are regulated by hormones.

VI. The volume and composition of body fluid must be regulated.
   A. The body has two main fluid compartments.
   B. Fluid intake must equal fluid output.
   C. Electrolyte balance and fluid balance are interdependent.
   D. Electrolytes serve vital functions.

VII. Acid-base balance must be maintained.

Learning Objectives

After you have studied this chapter, you should be able to:

1. Identify the principal metabolic waste products and the organs that excrete them.

2. Summarize the functions of the urinary system in maintaining homeostasis.

3. Label a diagram of the urinary system and give the function of each structure.

4. Describe the structure and function of a nephron. (Be able to label a diagram of a nephron.)

5. Trace a drop of filtrate from glomerulus to urethra, listing in sequence each structure through which it passes.

6. Describe the process of urine formation and give the composition of urine.

7. Summarize the regulation of urine volume including the actions of antidiuretic hormone (ADH), renin, aldosterone, angiotensin II, and atrial natriuretic peptide (ANP).

8. Identify the fluid compartments of the body.

9. Summarize the mechanisms that regulate fluid intake and fluid output.

10. Define electrolyte balance and identify the functions of five major electrolytes.

11. Describe the mechanisms responsible for sodium and potassium homeostasis.

12. Describe three mechanisms for maintaining acid-base balance.

STUDY QUESTIONS

Within each category, fill in the blanks with the correct response.

INTRODUCTION

Elimination   Excretion   Urinary   Excesses   Homeostatic   Water

1. The _____ system helps regulate the volume and composition of body fluids.

2. _____ is an excellent solvent.

3. Regardless of how much of it you eat or drink, the fluid and salt content of your body must be kept within

    _____ limits.

4. The body must replace water and salt losses and excrete _____.

5. _____ is defined as the discharge of metabolic byproducts and wastes, as well as excess solutes and other substances, from the body.

6. Excretion is different from _____, the discharge of undigested or unabsorbed food from the digestive tract.

I. METABOLIC WASTE PRODUCTS INCLUDE WATER, CARBON DIOXIDE, AND NITROGENOUS WASTES

Ammonia   Liver   Nitrogenous wastes   Kidneys   Lungs
Sweat glands   Urine   Hemoglobin   Uric acid   Nitrogen   Urea

1. The principal metabolic byproducts are water, carbon dioxide, _____, amino acids, and nucleic acids.

2. Amino acids and nucleic acids contain _____.

3. The amino group is chemically converted to _____, which is then converted to

    _____.

4. _____ is formed from the breakdown of nucleic acids.

5. Urea and uric acid are transported from the liver to the _____ by the circulatory system.

6. _____ in the skin excrete 5% to 10% of all metabolic wastes.

7. Sweat contains the same substances as _____, but is much more dilute.

8. The _____ excrete carbon dioxide and water (in the form of water vapor).

9. The _____ excretes bile pigments, which are products of the breakdown of

_____.

II.   THE URINARY SYSTEM HAS MANY REGULATORY FUNCTIONS

Blood   Erythropoietin   Renin   Body fluids   Excretes   Urine

1. The urinary system maintains homeostasis by adjusting the salt and water content of the

_____.

2. The urinary system _____ metabolic waste products such as urea.

3. The urinary system regulates the acid-base (pH) level of the _____ and other

_____.

4. The urinary system secretes the enzyme _____, which is important in regulating blood pressure.

5. The urinary system secretes the hormone _____, which regulates production of red blood cells.

III.   THE URINARY SYSTEM CONSISTS OF THE KIDNEYS, URINARY BLADDER, AND THEIR DUCTS

Bladder   Ureters   Urinary bladder   Kidneys   Urethra   Urine

1. The principal organs of the urinary system are the paired _____, which play a vital role in regulating the volume and consumption of body fluid.

2. The kidneys remove metabolic byproducts and wastes from the blood and produce

_____.

3. From the kidneys, urine is conducted to the urinary _____ by the paired

_____.

4. The single _____ temporarily stores urine.

5. Eventually, urine is discharged from the body through the single _____.

A. The Kidneys Consist of a Cortex and Medulla

Calyx	**Kidney**	**Renal artery**	**Renal pelvis**	**Major calyx**	**Renal capsule**
Cortex	**Hilus**	**Renal vein**	**Medulla**	**Renal papilla**	**Retroperitoneal**

1. The kidneys are located behind the peritoneum lining the abdominal cavity, and so are described as

   _____.

2. Each kidney receives blood from a _____, and is drained by a

   _____.

3. Each _____ resembles a large, dark-red lima bean about the size of a fist.

4. The ureters and blood vessels connect with the kidney at its _____, the notch on its medial border.

5. Covering the kidney is a strong capsule of connective tissue, the _____.

6. The kidney consists of an outer renal _____ and an inner renal

   _____.

7. The tip of each renal pyramid is called a _____.

8. Urine passes from a collecting duct through a renal papilla and into a small tube called a minor

   _____.

9. Several minor calyces unite to form a _____.

10. The major calyces join to form a large cavity, the _____.

11. Place the correct number next to each choice to indicate the proper sequence.

    _____ Calyx

    _____ Renal pelvis

    _____ Ureter

    _____ Collecting duct

    _____ Renal papilla

B.   The Nephrons Are the Functional Units of the Kidney

Afferent arteriole	**Corpuscle**	**Tubule**	**Efferent arteriole**	**Urine**
Bowman's capsule	**Filtrate**	**Nephrons**	**Peritubular**	
Collecting ducts	**Glomerulus**	**Blood**	**Juxtaglomerular**	

1.   Each kidney contains more than 1 million microscopic units called _____.

2.   Nephrons filter the blood and produce _____.

3.   Blood is filtered in the renal _____, then the filtered fluid, referred to as the

_____, passes through the long renal _____.

4.   As the filtrate moves through the renal tubule, substances needed by the body are returned to the

_____. Waste products, excess water, and other solutes that are not needed by the

body pass into the _____ and exit as urine.

5.   Each renal corpuscle consists of a network of capillaries, the _____, surrounded by a

cuplike structure known as _____, or glomerular capsule.

6.   Blood from the renal artery flows into the glomerulus through a small _____, and

leaves the glomerulus through an _____.

7.   The _____ capillaries surround the renal tubule.

8.   Part of the distal convoluted tubule curves upward and contacts the afferent arteriole. The cells that make

this contact form the _____ apparatus.

9.   Place the correct number next to each choice to indicate the proper sequence.

_____   Loop of Henle

_____   Collecting duct

_____   Bowman's capsule

_____   Distal convoluted tubule

_____   Proximal convoluted tubule

C. Urine Is Transported by Ducts and Stored in the Bladder

Bladder   Prostate   Urinary bladder   Penis   Ureters   Vagina   Peristaltic   Urethra

1. Urine passes from the kidneys through the paired _____.

2. Urine is forced along through the ureter by _____ contractions.

3. The _____ is a temporary storage sac for urine.

4. When urine leaves the bladder, it flows through the _____, a duct leading to the outside of the body.

5. In the male, the urethra is long and passes through the _____ gland and the

   _____.

6. In the female, the urethra is short and is found just above the opening into the

   _____.

7. _____ infections are more common in females than males because the long male urethra is a barrier to bacterial invasion.

D. Urination Empties the Bladder

External urethral sphincter   Nervous system   Urination reflex   Micturition   Urinate

1. Urination, or _____, is the process of emptying the bladder and expelling urine.

2. The _____ contracts smooth muscle fibers in the bladder wall and also relaxes the internal urethral sphincter.

3. When the time and place are appropriate, the _____ is voluntarily relaxed, allowing urination to occur.

4. Voluntary control of urination cannot be exerted by an immature _____.

5. Most babies under the age of about 2.5 years automatically _____ every time the bladder fills.

IV. URINE IS PRODUCED BY FILTRATION, REABSORPTION, AND SECRETION

Glomerular   Tubular reabsorption   Tubular secretion

1. Urine is produced by a combination of three processes: _____ filtration,

   _____, and _____.

A.   Glomerular Filtration Is Not Selective With Regard to Small Molecules and Ions

Body   **Glucose**   **Blood cells**   **Glomerular filtration**   **Amino acids**
Kidney   **Proteins**   **Blood plasma**   **Glomerular filtrate**

1.   The first step in urine production is _____.

2.   Blood flow through glomerular capillaries is at much higher pressure than in other capillaries. As a result,

     more plasma is filtered in the _____ and a large amount of

     _____ is produced.

3.   Glomerular filtrate consists of _____ containing ions and small, dissolved molecules.

4.   Substances needed by the body, such as _____, _____, and
     salts are present in the glomerular filtrate.

5.   When _____ or _____ appear in the urine, they are signals of
     a problem with glomerular filtration.

6.   Every 4 minutes the kidneys receive a volume of blood equal to the volume of blood in the

     _____.

B.   Tubular Reabsorption Is Highly Selective

Ducts   Selective   Urine   Renal tubules   Tubular reabsorption

1.   About 99% of glomerular filtrate is returned to the blood by _____.

2.   Tubular reabsorption is the job of the _____ and collecting

     _____.

3.   Unlike glomerular filtration, tubular reabsorption is highly _____.

4.   Wastes, surplus salts, and excess water are kept as part of the filtrate and are excreted as

     _____.

C.   Some Substances Are Secreted From the Blood Into the Filtrate

Creatinine   Penicillin   Tubular secretion   Homeostatic   Renal tubules

1.   In _____, certain substances are actively transported from the blood in the

     peritubular capillaries into the filtrate in the _____.

2. Potassium, hydrogen ions, ammonium ions, and some organic ions such as the waste product

_____ are secreted into the filtrate.

3. Secretion of hydrogen ions is an important _____ mechanism for regulating the pH of the blood.

4. Certain drugs such as _____ are also removed from the blood by secretion.

D.   Urine Consists Mainly of Water

Ammonia   Renal pelvis   Urine   Bacterial action   Salts   Water   Nitrogen wastes   Sterile

1. By the time the filtrate reaches the _____, its composition has been carefully adjusted.

2. The adjusted filtrate is called _____.

3. Urine is composed of about 96% _____, 2.5% _____, 1.5%

_____, and traces of other substances.

4. Healthy urine is _____, and has been used to wash battlefield wounds when clean water was not available.

5. Urine rapidly decomposes when exposed to _____, forming ammonia and other products.

6. It is the _____ in urine that causes diaper rash in infants.

V.   URINE VOLUME AND COMPOSITION ARE REGULATED BY HORMONES

ADH   Dehydrate   Reabsorption   Aldosterone   Osmotic pressure
Diuretics   Kidney   Greater   Hypothalamus   Diabetes insipidus

1. The _____ receives information about the state of the blood indirectly.

2. When fluid intake is low, the body begins to _____.

3. When the volume of blood decreases, the concentration of dissolved salts is _____,

causing an increase in the _____ of the blood.

4. Specialized receptors in the _____ are sensitive to changes in the osmotic pressure.

5. The hormone _____ regulates the excretion of water by the kidneys.

6. When the pituitary gland does not produce enough ADH, water is not efficiently reabsorbed from the ducts. This results in the production of a large volume of urine. This condition is called

   _____.

7. The hormone _____ acts on the kidney tubules, increasing the reabsorption of sodium.

8. Coffee, tea, and alcoholic beverages contain chemicals called _____ that increase urine volume.

9. Diuretics inhibit _____ of water.

VI.   THE VOLUME AND COMPOSITION OF BODY FLUID MUST BE REGULATED

Water   Chemical reactions   Lymph   Blood plasma   Interstitial fluid   Transport

1. The human body is about 60% _____ by weight.

2. Body fluids such as _____, _____, and

   _____ consist mainly of water.

3. All of the _____ in the body take place in a watery medium.

4. Water is used to _____ materials throughout the body.

A.   The Body Has Two Main Fluid Compartments

Blood pressure   Intracellular   Volume   Cells   Lymphatic   Extracellular   Osmotic

1. Body fluid is distributed in two principal compartments: the _____ compartment

   and the _____ compartment.

2. About two-thirds of the body fluid is found within _____.

3. Fluid constantly moves from one compartment to another. However, in a healthy person, the

   _____ of fluid in each compartment remains about the same.

4. The movement of fluid from one compartment to another depends on _____ and

   _____ concentration.

5. Excess interstitial fluid is returned to the blood by the _____ system.

B. Fluid Intake Must Equal Fluid Output

Dehydration   Hypothalamus   Kidneys   Thirst center   Fluid output   Ingested   Metabolism

1. Normally, fluid intake equals _____.

2. The average daily fluid intake is about 2500 ml, most of which is _____ in the foods we eat and liquids we drink.

3. Water is produced during cellular _____.

4. Fluid is excreted primarily by the _____.

5. When fluid output is greater than fluid intake, _____ occurs.

6. Fluid intake is regulated by the _____.

7. Dehydration causes increased osmotic pressure which stimulates the _____ in the hypothalamus.

C. Electrolyte Balance and Fluid Balance Are Interdependent

Anions   Electrolytes   Nonelectrolytes   Cations   Glucose   Urea   Electrolyte balance   Ions

1. Among the most important components of body fluids are _____.

2. Electrolytes are compounds such as inorganic salts, acids, and bases that form _____ in solution.

3. Most organic compounds dissolved in the body fluid are _____—compounds that do not form ions.

4. Examples of nonelectrolytes in the body fluid are _____ and

    _____.

5. Positively charged ions are referred to as _____.

6. Negatively charged ions are referred to as _____.

7. When the amounts of the various electrolytes taken into the body equal the amounts lost, the body is in

    _____.

D.   Electrolytes Serve Vital Functions

Heart failure	**Urine**	**Aldosterone**	**Magnesium**	**Acid-base (pH)**
Phosphate	**Water**	**Chloride**	**Muscle**	**Potassium**
Coma	**Nervous**	**Sodium**	**Osmotic pressure**	

1.   About 90% of the extracellular cations are _____ ions.

2.   Sodium ions are needed to transmit impulses in _____ and

_____ tissue.

3.   Severe sodium depletion may result in circulatory shock and _____.

4.   Sodium ion concentration is adjusted mainly by regulating the amount of _____ in
the body.

5.   _____ stimulates the distal convoluted tubules and collecting ducts to increase their
reabsorption of sodium ions.

6.   Most of the cations in the intracellular fluid are _____ ions.

7.   Potassium ions help regulate _____ levels.

8.   A high potassium ion concentration can weaken the heart and lead to death from arrhythmia, or

_____.

9.   Loss of potassium ions in the _____ brings the potassium concentration in the body
back to normal.

10.   _____ ions are the most abundant intracellular anions.

11.   _____ ions are the most abundant extracellular anions.

12.   Chloride ions help regulate differences in _____ between fluid compartments and are
also important in pH balance.

13.   _____ ions are important in development of bones and teeth and play a role in
neural transmission and muscle contraction.

VII.   ACID-BASE BALANCE MUST BE MAINTAINED

Acid-base	**Higher**	**Bicarbonate**	**Lower**	**Respiratory acidosis**
Protein	**Acidity**	**Acidosis**	**Neutral**	**Respiratory alkalosis**
Alkalinity	**Basic**	**PH**	**Alkalosis**	**Chemical buffer**
Blood	**Hemoglobin**	**Phosphate**		

1.   _____ balance depends on the concentration of hydrogen ions.

2. _____ is a measurement of the hydrogen ion concentration of a solution.

3. A _____ pH is 7.

4. Lower pH values indicate a _____ hydrogen ion concentration or a higher

_____.

5. Higher pH values indicate a _____ hydrogen ion concentration or greater

_____.

6. An alkaline solution is also referred to as _____.

7. _____ and most other body fluids are slightly alkaline.

8. The term _____ refers to any condition in which the hydrogen ion concentration of plasma is elevated above the homeostatic range.

9. _____ is any condition in which the hydrogen ion concentration is below the homeostatic range.

10. A _____ is a substance that minimizes changes in pH when an acid or base is added to a solution.

11. The main buffering systems in the body are the _____ buffer system, the

_____ buffer system, and the _____ buffer systems.

12. _____ is an example of a protein that is a very effective buffer.

13. _____ develops when carbon dioxide is produced more rapidly than it is excreted by the lungs.

14. _____ occurs when the respiratory system excretes carbon dioxide more quickly than it is produced.

Labeling Exercise

Please fill in the correct labels for Figure 16-1.

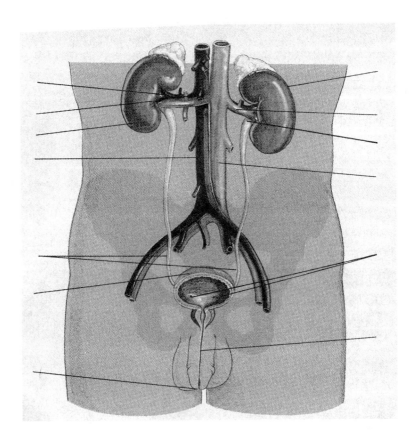

Figure 16-1

Labeling Exercise

Please fill in the correct labels for Figure 16-2.

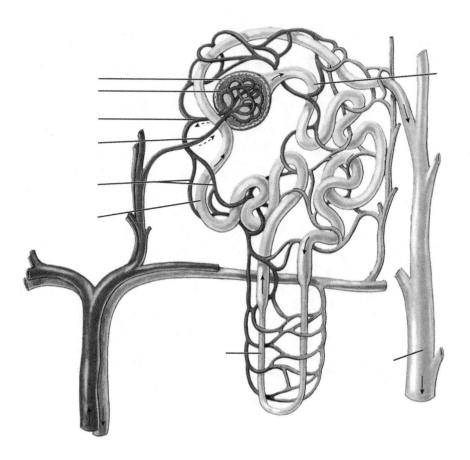

Figure 16-2

CHAPTER TEST

Select the correct response.

1. Which of the following is not a metabolic waste product?
   a. water
   b. glucose
   c. wastes that contain nitrogen
   d. carbon dioxide

2. Organs that function in waste disposal include the
   a. urinary system.
   b. skin.
   c. lungs.
   d. all of the above.

3. Organs of the urinary system include all but the
   a. kidneys.
   b. spleen.
   c. ureters.
   d. urethra.

4. The correct order of urine flow through the urinary system is
   a. kidney, ureter, bladder, and urethra.
   b. bladder, ureter, kidney, and urethra.
   c. kidney, urethra, bladder, and ureter.
   d. bladder, urethra, kidney, and ureter.

5. Urine flows through the following structures in which sequence?
    a. renal papilla, collecting duct, calyx, renal pelvis, and ureter
    b. collecting duct, renal papilla, calyx, renal pelvis, and ureter
    c. renal pelvis, renal papilla, calyx, collecting duct, and ureter
    d. calyx, renal pelvis, renal papilla, collecting duct, and ureter

6. Filtrate flows through the following structures in which sequence?
    a. loop of Henle, Bowman's capsule, proximal convoluted tubule, collecting duct, and distal convoluted tubule
    b. Bowman's capsule, proximal convoluted tubules, loop of Henle, collecting duct, distal convoluted tubule
    c. Bowman's capsule, proximal convoluted tubules, loop of Henle, distal convoluted tubule, collecting duct
    d. Bowman's capsule, proximal convoluted tubules, collecting duct, distal convoluted tubule, loop of Henle

7. The average adult urinary bladder can stretch so it can hold up to _____ of urine.
    a. 100 ml
    b. 800 ml
    c. 100 L
    d. 800 L

8. Which of the following is not a function of the kidney?
    a. produces renin
    b. produces aldosterone
    c. produces erythropoietin
    d. helps regulate the pH of the blood

9. Urine production involves all but
    a. glomerular filtration.
    b. tubular reabsorption.
    c. renal acidosis.
    d. tubular secretion.

10. The first step in urine production is
    a. tubular reabsorption.
    b. glomerular filtration.
    c. tubular secretion.
    d. Bowman's capsule.

11. Which of the following is not a factor that contributes to the large amount of glomerular filtrate?
    a. The afferent arteriole is smaller in diameter than the efferent arteriole.
    b. The highly coiled glomerular capillaries provide a large surface area for filtration.
    c. The glomerular capillaries are greatly permeable.
    d. Blood flow through glomerular capillaries is at much higher pressure than in other capillaries.

12. _____ is a selective process.
    a. Tubular reabsorption
    b. Glomerular filtration
    c. Tubular secretion
    d. a and c only

13. Urine consists mainly of
    a. blood.
    b. sugar.
    c. water.
    d. salt.

14. Dehydration can result from
    a. profuse sweating.
    b. not drinking enough fluids.
    c. vomiting or diarrhea.
    d. all of the above.

15. Low sodium ion concentration can cause all but which of the following?
    a. headache
    b. high blood pressure
    c. low blood pressure
    d. mental confusion

16. Calcium ions are essential in which of the following?
    a. blood clotting
    b. regulation of pH
    c. muscle contraction
    d. both a and c

17. Acid ingested in foods, but not neutralized by the ingestion of alkaline foods, is neutralized by all but which of the following?
    a. muscular system
    b. respiratory system
    c. chemical buffers
    d. kidneys

Chapter

17

REPRODUCTION

■ ■ ■

Outline

Introduction
I. The male produces sperm.
  A. The testes produce sperm and hormones.
  B. The conducting tubes transport sperm.
  C. The accessory glands produce semen.
  D. The penis delivers sperm into the female reproductive tract.
  E. Hormones regulate male reproduction.
II. The female produces ova and incubates the embryo.
  A. The ovaries produce ova and hormones.
  B. The uterine tubes transport ova.
  C. The uterus incubates the embryo.
  D. The vagina functions in sexual intercourse, menstruation, and birth.
  E. The external genital structures are the vulva.
F. The breasts contain the mammary glands.
G. Hormones regulate female reproduction.
III. Fertilization is the fusion of sperm and ovum.
IV. The zygote gives rise to the new individual.
  A. The embryo develops in the wall of the uterus.
  B. Prenatal development requires about 266 days.
  C. The birth process includes labor and delivery.
  D. Multiple births may be fraternal or identical.
V. The human life cycle extends from fertilization to death.

Learning Objectives

After you have studied this chapter, you should be able to:

1. Label a diagram of the male reproductive system and describe the functions of each structure.
2. Trace the passage of sperm from the tubules in the testes through the conducting tubes, describing changes that may occur along the way.
3. Describe the actions of the male gonadotropic hormones and of testosterone.
4. Label diagrams of internal and external female reproductive organs and describe their structure and functions.
5. Trace the development of an ovum and its passage through the female reproductive system.
6. Describe the principal events of the menstrual cycle and summarize the interactions of hormones that regulate the cycle.
7. Describe the process of fertilization.
8. Summarize the course of development from fertilization to birth.
9. Describe the functions of the amnion and placenta.
10. Identify the three stages of the birth process.
11. List the stages of human development from fertilization to death.

STUDY QUESTIONS

Within each category, fill in the blanks with the correct response.

INTRODUCTION

Gametes   Gonads   Lactation   Reproduction

1. _____ involves several processes including preparation of the female body for pregnancy, sexual intercourse, fertilization, pregnancy, and lactation.

2. Eggs and sperm are specialized sex cells called _____.

3. The mother's production of milk for nourishing her infant is called _____.

4. The sex glands are referred to as _____.

I.   THE MALE PRODUCES SPERM

Egg   Scrotum   Sperm   Penis   Sex   Testes

1. The male's function in reproduction is to produce _____ cells and deliver them into the female reproductive tract.

2. When a sperm combines with a(n) _____, it contributes half the genes of the

   offspring and determines the _____ of the baby.

3. Male reproductive structures include the _____ and _____, the conducting tubes that lead from the testes to the outside of the body, the accessory glands and the

   _____.

A.   The Testes Produce Sperm and Hormones

Inguinal	**Scrotum**	**Inguinal hernia**	**Spermatogenesis**
Testes	**Sperm**	**Chromosomes**	**Seminiferous**

1. In the adult male, millions of sperm cells are manufactured each day within the paired male gonads, the

   _____.

2. The _____ tubules are the sperm cell factories, and they also produce male hormones.

3. The process of sperm production is called _____.

4. During fertilization, one set of 23 _____ is contributed by the mother's ovum and the other set by the father's sperm.

5. The mature _____ is a tiny, elongated cell with a tail (flagellum) that is used for moving toward an egg.

6. The testes develop in the abdominal cavity of the male embryo. About 2 months before birth, they descend

    into the _____, a skin-covered sac suspended from the groin.

7. As the testes descend, they move through the _____ canals.

8. Straining the abdominal muscles by lifting a very heavy object may result in a tear in the inguinal wall, through which a loop of intestine can bulge into the scrotum. This is called a(n)

    _____.

B.   The Conducting Tubes Transport Sperm

Ejaculatory   Sperm   Urethra   Vas deferens   Epididymis   Spermatic cord   Urine

1. From the tubules inside the testes, sperm pass into a large, coiled tube, the _____.

2. The epididymis empties into a straight tube, the _____, or sperm duct.

3. The vas deferens passes from the scrotum through the inguinal canal as part of the

    _____.

4. The vas deferens is joined by the duct from the seminal vesicles to become the

    _____ duct.

5. The ejaculatory duct passes through the prostate gland, and then opens into the

    _____.

6. The single urethra, which conducts both _____ and _____, passes through the penis to the outside of the body.

7. Place the correct number next to each choice to indicate the proper sequence.

    _____ Vas deferens

    _____ Urethra

    _____ Tubules in the testis

    _____ Epididymis

    _____ Ejaculatory duct

C.   The Accessory Glands Produce Semen

Bulbourethral   Prostate   Sperm cells   Ejaculation   Semen   Sterile

1. _____ is a thick, whitish fluid consisting of sperm cells suspended in secretions of the accessory glands.

2. The single _____ gland surrounds the urethra as the urethra emerges from the urinary bladder.

3. The _____, or Cowper's, glands are about the size and shape of two peas, one on each side of the urethra.

4. Semen is discharged from the penis during _____.

5. Semen consists of about 200 million _____ suspended in the secretions of the accessory glands.

6. Men with fewer than 20 million sperm/ml of semen usually are _____.

D.   The Penis Delivers Sperm Into the Female Reproductive Tract

Circumcision   Erect   Prepuce   Sinusoids   Corpus   Glans   Reflex   Ejaculation   Penis   Shaft

1. The _____ is the male copulatory organ.

2. The penis consists of a long _____ that enlarges to form an expanded tip, the

   _____.

3. Part of the loose-fitting skin of the penis folds down and covers the proximal portion of the glans, forming a

   cuff called the _____, or foreskin.

4. The foreskin is removed during _____.

5. Under the skin, the penis consists of three cylinders of spongy tissue called erectile tissue. Each cylinder,

   referred to as a _____, contains blood vessels called _____.

6. When the male becomes excited, spongy tissue in the penis fills with blood and the penis becomes

   _____.

7. When the level of sexual excitement reaches a peak, _____ occurs.

8. Both erection and ejaculation are _____ actions.

E.   Hormones Regulate Male Reproduction

Androgens   **Hypothalamus**   **Puberty**   **Follicle-stimulating hormone (FSH)**
Secondary   **Testosterone**   **Gonadotropic**   **Luteinizing hormone (LH)**
Primary   **Development**   **Negative feedback**

1. Male hormones are referred to as _____.

2. Interstitial cells produce the principal male hormone _____.

3. Testosterone is the hormone responsible for the _____ of both primary and secondary sex characteristics in the male.

4. _____ sex characteristics include the growth and activity of the reproductive structures, including the penis and scrotum.

5. _____ sex characteristics include deepening of the voice; muscle development; and growth of pubic, facial, and underarm hair.

6. _____ is the period of sexual maturation that typically begins between ages 10–12 years, and continues until ages 16–18 years.

7. At puberty, the _____ begins to secrete gonadotropin-releasing hormones (GnRH) that stimulate the anterior lobe of the pituitary gland to secrete _____ hormones.

8. The gonadotropic hormone, _____, stimulates sperm production.

9. The gonadotropic hormone, _____, stimulates the testes to secrete testosterone.

10. Reproductive hormone concentrations are regulated by _____ mechanisms.

Labeling Exercise

Please fill in the correct labels for Figure 17-1.

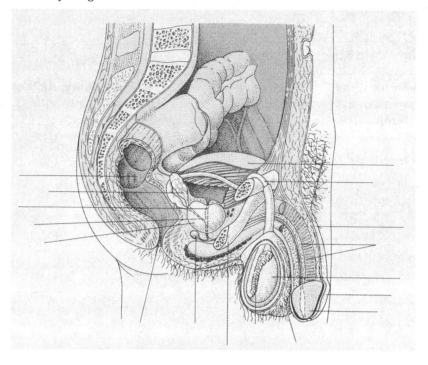

Figure 17-1

Labeling Exercise

Please fill in the correct labels for Figure 17-2.

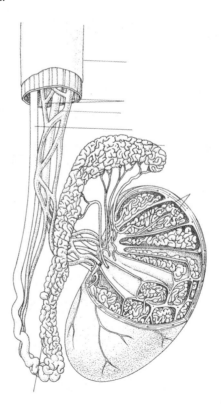

Figure 17-2

II.   THE FEMALE PRODUCES OVA AND INCUBATES THE EMBRYO

Menstrual cycle   Ovaries   Uterus   Ova   Sperm   Vagina

1. The female reproductive system produces _____, and receives the penis and the

    _____ released from it during sexual intercourse.

2. Much of the activity of the female reproductive system centers about the _____, the
    monthly preparation for possible pregnancy.

3. The _____ produce ova and female hormones.

4. The _____ is the incubator for the developing child.

5. The _____ receives the penis during intercourse and serves as a birth canal.

A.   The Ovaries Produce Ova and Hormones

Corpus luteum	**Graafian**	**Ovaries**	**Estrogen**	**Oogenesis**	**Ovulation**
Female hormones	**Ova**	**Progesterone**	**Follicle**	**Ovarian**	**Puberty**

1. The paired _____ are the female gonads.

2. The ovaries produce _____ and the female sex hormones,

    _____ and _____.

3. The _____ ligament anchors the medial end of the ovary to the uterus.

4. The process of ovum development is called _____.

5. The ovum and its surrounding sac make up a _____.

6. With the onset of _____, a few follicles develop each month.

7. Cells of the follicle secrete _____, called estrogens.

8. Mature follicles are called _____ follicles.

9. During _____, the ovum is ejected through the wall of the ovary and into the pelvic
    cavity.

10. The part of the follicle that remains behind in the ovary develops into an important temporary endocrine

    structure, the _____.

B. The Uterine Tubes Transport Ova

Oviduct Fimbriae Uterus Fallopian Ovum Zygote Fertilization Pelvic

1. Each uterine tube, also called the _____ or _____ tube, is about 12 cm long.

2. The free end of the fallopian tube is shaped like a funnel and has long, fingerlike projections called

    _____.

3. During ovulation, the mature ovum is released into the _____ cavity.

4. Action of the cilia in the lining of the uterine tube helps move the ovum toward the

    _____.

5. Normally, _____ takes place in the upper third of the uterine tube.

6. The fertilized egg, or _____, begins its development as it is moved along toward the uterus.

7. If fertilization does not occur, the _____ degenerates in the uterine tube.

C. The Uterus Incubates the Embryo

Cervix Endometrium Papanicolaou (Pap) Corpus Fundus Uterus Embryo Menstruation

1. Each month during a woman's reproductive life, the _____, or womb, prepares for possible pregnancy.

2. When pregnancy occurs, the uterus serves as the incubator for the developing _____.

3. If pregnancy does not occur, the inner lining of the uterus sloughs off each month and is discarded. This

    process is called _____.

4. The main portion of the uterus is its _____, or body.

5. The rounded part of the uterus above the level of the entrance of the uterine tubes is the

    _____.

6. The lower, narrow portion of the uterus is the _____, which projects into the vagina.

7. The uterus is lined by a mucous membrane, the _____.

8. The routine _____ test can usually detect cervical cancer.

D.   The Vagina Functions in Sexual Intercourse, Menstruation, and Birth

Cervix   Endometrium   Fornices   Vagina   Collapsed   Enlarging   Rugae

1. The _____ functions as the sexual organ that receives the penis during sexual intercourse.

2. The vagina serves as an exit through which the discarded _____ is discharged during menstruation.

3. The vagina surrounds the end of the _____.

4. The recesses formed between the vaginal wall and the cervix are called _____.

5. The vagina is normally _____ so that its walls touch each other. Two ridges run along the anterior and posterior walls and there are numerous _____, or folds.

6. During sexual intercourse, or during childbirth, the rugae straighten out, greatly

    _____ the vagina.

E.   The External Genital Structures Are the Vulva

Bartholin's	**Labia majora**	**Vulva**	**Urethra**	**Vagina**	**Clinical perineum**
Clitoris	**Mons pubis**	**Vestibule**	**Hymen**	**Puberty**	**Labia minora**

1. The term _____ refers to the external female genital structures.

2. The _____ is a mound of fatty tissue that covers the pubic symphysis.

3. At _____, the mons pubis becomes covered by coarse pubic hair.

4. The paired _____ are folds of skin that pass form the mons pubis to the region behind the vaginal opening.

5. Two thin folds of skin, the _____ are located just within the labia majora.

6. The _____ is a small structure that corresponds to the male glans and is a main focus of sexual sensation in the female.

7. The space enclosed by the labia minora is the _____.

8. Two openings can be seen in the vestibule—the opening of the _____ anteriorly, and the opening of the _____ posteriorly.

9. A thin ring of mucous membrane, the _____, surrounds the entrance to the vagina.

10. Two small _____ glands open on each side of the vaginal opening.

11. The region between the vagina and anus is referred to as the _____.

F. The Breasts Contain the Mammary Glands

Breasts	Milk	Prolactin	Colostrum	Ligaments of Cooper
Lymphatic	Nipple	Lactation	Oxytocin	Mammography

1. The breasts function in _____—production and release of milk for nourishment of the baby.

2. The _____ overlie the pectoral muscles and are attached to them by connective tissue.

3. Fibrous bands of tissue called _____ firmly connect the breasts to the skin.

4. The mammary glands, located within the breasts, produce _____.

5. The _____ consists of smooth muscle that can contract to make the nipple erect in response to sexual stimuli.

6. For the first few days after childbirth, the mammary glands produce a fluid called

_____, which contains protein and lactose but little fat.

7. After childbirth, _____ stimulates milk production.

8. _____ stimulates ejection of milk from the glands into the ducts.

9. Breast cancer often spreads to the _____ system.

10. _____, a soft-tissue radiological study of the breast, is helpful in detecting very small lesions that might not be identified by routine examination.

G. Hormones Regulate Female Reproduction

Menarche	Menstruation	Puberty	Estrogens	Estrogen replacement
Menopause	Ovulation	LH	Progesterone	Menstrual cycle

1. The ovaries secrete estrogens and _____.

2. Like testosterone in the male, _____ are responsible for the growth of sex organs at puberty and for the development of secondary sex characteristics.

3. In the female, _____ typically begins between 10 and 12 years and continues until 14 to 16 years.

4. _____ is the first menstrual period, and usually occurs between 12 and 14 years.

5. During the _____, estrogens stimulate the growth of follicles and the endometrium.

6. _____ typically occurs about 14 days before the next menstrual cycle begins.

7. During _____, the thickened endometrium of the uterus sloughs off.

8. _____ is necessary for final maturation of the follicle, ovulation, and development of the corpus luteum.

9. At about age 50 years, a woman enters _____—the time when ova are no longer produced and the woman is no longer fertile.

10. _____ therapy relieves many of the symptoms of menopause.

Labeling Exercise

Please fill in the correct labels for Figure 17-3.

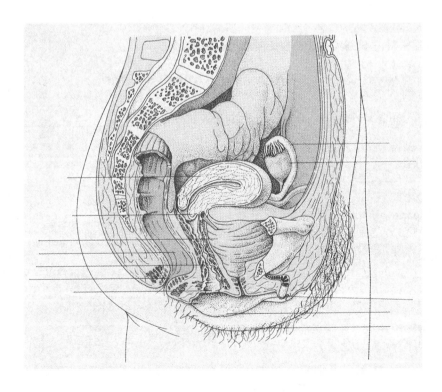

Figure 17-3

Labeling Exercise

Please fill in the correct labels for Figure 17-4.

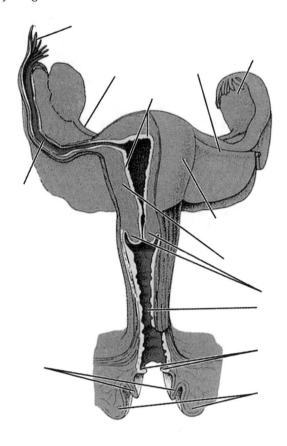

Figure 17-4

III. FERTILIZATION IS THE FUSION OF SPERM AND OVUM

Ejaculation Follicle Ovum Zygote Fertilization Ovulation Uterus

1. When sperm are released in the vagina, some find their way into the _____ and uterine tubes.

2. _____ is the fusion of the sperm and the egg.

3. Large numbers of sperm are necessary to penetrate the _____ cells surrounding the ovum (egg).

4. As soon as one sperm penetrates the _____, no other sperm is able to get into the ovum.

5. Sperm and ovum fuse to form a fertilized egg, or _____.

6. After _____, sperm remain viable for only about 48 hours.

7. The ovum remains fertile for approximately 24 hours after _____.

IV. THE ZYGOTE GIVES RISE TO THE NEW INDIVIDUAL

Cilia   Embryo   Uterine tube   Uterus   Zygote

1. The _____ contains all of the genetic information necessary to produce a complete individual.

2. The zygote divides to form a(n) _____ that is composed of two cells.

3. As the first cell divisions take place, the embryo is slowly moved along the _____

toward the uterus by the action of _____.

4. By the time the embryo reaches the _____ on the 5th day of development, it is a tiny cluster of about 32 cells.

A. The Embryo Develops in the Wall of the Uterus

Amnion   Placenta   Umbilical cord   Human chorionic gonadotropin (hCG)
Blood   Uterus   Fetal   Progesterone

1. On about the seventh day of the development, the embryo begins to implant itself in the wall of the

_____.

2. Several _____ membranes develop around the embryo. They help protect, nourish, and support the developing embryo.

3. The _____ is a membrane that forms a sac around the embryo.

4. The _____ is the organ of exchange between the mother and the embryo.

5. Wastes from the embryo move through the placenta and into the mother's _____.

6. During pregnancy, the corpus luteum and the placenta secrete _____.

7. The placenta produces a hormone called _____, which signals the corpus luteum to increase in size and to release large amounts of estrogens and progesterone.

8. The stalk of tissue that connects the embryo with the placenta is the _____.

B. Prenatal Development Requires About 266 Days

Brain   Menstrual period   Cerebrum   Lanugo   Premature
Fetus   Fetal movements   Limb buds   Spinal cord

1. Obstetricians typically count from the onset of the mother's last _____, and consider an average pregnancy 280 days (40 weeks).

2. The _____ and _____ are among the first organs to develop.

3. Small mounds of tissue called _____ can be seen by the end of the first month, and slowly lengthen and form the limbs.

4. After the second month, the embryo is referred to as a(n) _____.

5. The mother usually becomes aware of _____ by about 5 months of development.

6. During the 7th month, the _____ grows rapidly and develops convolutions (folds).

7. Most of the body of the fetus is covered by downy hair called _____.

8. If a baby is born before 37 weeks, it is considered _____.

C. The Birth Process Includes Labor and Delivery

Afterbirth	Dilated	Parturition	Amnion	Effaced	Placenta
Amniotic	First stage	Second stage	Delivery	Labor	Third stage

1. Childbirth, or _____, includes labor and delivery.

2. _____ begins with a long series of involuntary contractions of the uterus.

3. During the _____ of labor, regular uterine contractions become more intense, rhythmic, and frequent.

4. During the first stage of labor, the cervix becomes _____ to about 10 cm, and

   becomes _____, or continuous with the uterine wall.

5. Rupture of the _____, with the release of the _____ fluid through the vagina may occur during the first stage of labor.

6. The _____ of labor begins when the cervix is fully dilated and ends with the

   _____ of the baby.

7. When the neonate emerges, it is still connected to the _____ by the umbilical cord.

8. During the _____ of labor, the placenta separates from the uterus and is expelled.

9. After delivery, the placenta is referred to as the _____; it is inspected for abnormalities and then discarded.

D. Multiple Births May Be Fraternal or Identical

Conjoined   Fraternal   Identical   Fertility   Genes

1. With the use of _____ drugs, multiple births have become much more common.

2. _____ twins develop when a woman ovulates two eggs and each is fertilized by a different sperm.

3. _____ twins develop when the tiny mass of cells that makes up the early embryo divides to form two independent groups of cells, and each develops into a baby.

4. Identical twins, developed from a single fertilized egg, thus have identical _____, and are indeed identical.

5. Rarely, two masses of embryonic cells do not separate completely and give rise to

_____ twins.

V. THE HUMAN LIFE CYCLE EXTENDS FROM FERTILIZATION TO DEATH

Adolescence	**Infancy**	**Childhood**	**Middle age**
Development	**Old age**	**Neonatal**	**Young adulthood**

1. _____ begins at fertilization and continues through the stages of the human life cycle until death.

2. The _____ period extends from birth to the end of the first month of postnatal life.

3. _____ follows the neonatal period and lasts until age 2 years.

4. _____, also a period of rapid growth and development, continues from infancy until adolescence.

5. _____ is the time of development between puberty and adulthood.

6. _____ extends from adolescence until about age 40.

7. _____ is usually considered to be the period between 40 and 65.

8. _____ begins after 65.

CHAPTER TEST

Select the correct response.

1. Reproduction involves several processes, including
   a. formation of gametes.
   b. preparation of the female body for pregnancy.
   c. sexual intercourse.
   d. all of the above.

2. Male reproductive structures include all but which of the following?
   a. testes
   b. ureters
   c. urethra
   d. vas deferens

3. The sequence of the path that sperm pass through is
   a. tubules in the testis, epididymis, vas deferens, urethra, and ejaculatory duct.
   b. tubules in the testis, vas deferens, epididymis, ejaculatory duct, and urethra.
   c. tubules in the testis, epididymis, vas deferens, ejaculatory duct, and urethra.
   d. epididymis, vas deferens, urethra, ejaculatory duct and tubules in the testes.

4. The _____ is the male copulatory organ.
   a. penis
   b. testis
   c. scrotum
   d. ureter

5. The _____ is removed during circumcision.
   a. shaft
   b. prepuce
   c. glans
   d. vas deferens

6. Primary sex characteristics in the male include
   a. growth of the penis and scrotum.
   b. growth and activity of internal reproductive structures.
   c. muscle development.
   d. both a and b.

7. Secondary sex characteristics in the male include all but which of the following?
   a. muscle development
   b. growth of the penis and scrotum
   c. growth of facial, pubic, and underarm hair
   d. deepening of the voice

8. A high concentration of _____ in the testes is required for spermatogenesis.
   a. testosterone
   b. estrogen
   c. progesterone
   d. cortisol

9. The organs of the female reproductive system include all but which of the following?
   a. ovaries
   b. uterine tubes
   c. urethra
   d. vagina

10. The _____ are the female gonads.
    a. uterine tubes
    b. ovaries
    c. breasts
    d. kidneys

11. In a normal pregnancy, the fetus develops in the
    a. ovaries.
    b. scrotum.
    c. uterus.
    d. uterine tubes.

12. The term *vulva* refers to the external female genital structures, which include the
    a. labia.
    b. vestibule.
    c. mons pubis.
    d. all of the above.

13. The mammary glands are located within the
    a. breasts.
    b. vagina.
    c. cervix.
    d. uterus.

14. Female secondary sex characteristics include all but which of the following?
    a. breast development
    b. broadening of the pelvis
    c. deepening of the voice
    d. distribution of fat and muscle that shape the female body

15. Although there is variation, a "typical" menstrual cycle is _____ days long.
    a. 3
    b. 7
    c. 28
    d. 45

16. During the menstrual cycle, ovulation occurs approximately _____ days before the next cycle begins.
    a. 7
    b. 14
    c. 28
    d. 36

17. By the fourth week of development, many organs in the fetus have begun to develop, including the _____.
    a. brain
    b. hands
    c. feet
    d. sex organs

18. The first stage of labor typically lasts
    a. 4–6 hours.
    b. 8–24 hours.
    c. 1–2 days.
    d. More than 2 days, but less than a week.

19. The umbilical cord connects the neonate to the
    a. mother's umbilicus.
    b. mother's vagina.
    c. placenta.
    d. hospital monitoring equipment.

20. When the cells that make up the early embryo divide completely to form two independent groups of cells, the resulting twins are
    a. fraternal.
    b. identical.
    c. conjoined.
    d. dizygotic.

CROSSWORD PUZZLE FOR CHAPTERS 16 AND 17

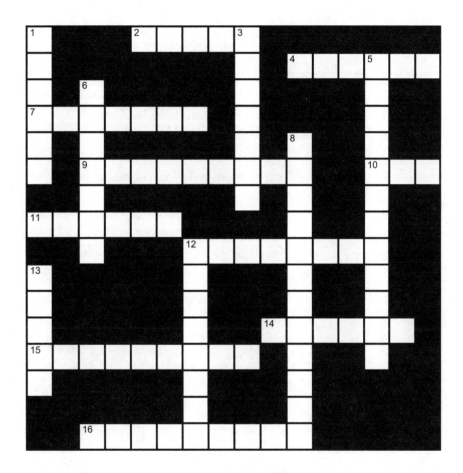

Across
2. Delivers sperm into the vagina
4. Organs that produce sperm
7. Female gonads
9. Stage at which menstrual cycle stops
10. Eggs
11. Portion of the uterus that projects into the vagina
12. Gland that surrounds the male urethra
14. Female sexual organ that receives the penis
15. Female sex hormones
16. Release of ovum from the ovary

Down
1. Fertilized egg
3. Sac that contains the testes
5. Male sex hormone
6. Glands located in the breasts
8. Monthly sloughing of the uterine lining
12. Organ through which the fetus receives nutrients
13. Membrane that partly blocks the entrance to the vagina

ANSWER KEY

∎ ∎ ∎

CHAPTER 1

STUDY QUESTIONS

INTRODUCING THE HUMAN BODY
1. Anatomy
2. Physiology
3. Adapted
4. Shape; Structure

I. THE BODY HAS SEVERAL LEVELS OF ORGANIZATION
1. Chemical
2. Atoms
3. Ion
4. Molecules
5. Water
6. Cells
7. Microscope
8. Organelles
9. Tissue
10. Functions
11. Muscle; Nervous; Connective; Epithelial
12. Organs
13. Organ
14. Organism

II. THE BODY IS COMPOSED OF INORGANIC COMPOUNDS AND ORGANIC COMPOUNDS
1. Inorganic
2. Organic
3. Carbohydrates
4. Steroids
5. Enzymes
6. Proteins
7. Amino
8. Nucleic
9. DNA
10. RNA

III. THE BODY SYSTEMS WORK TOGETHER TO MAINTAIN LIFE
1. Integumentary
2. Endocrine
3. Respiratory
4. Digestive
5. Muscular

IV. METABOLISM IS ESSENTIAL TO MAINTENANCE, GROWTH, AND REPAIR OF THE BODY
1. Metabolism
2. Anabolism; Catabolism
3. Breaking down
4. Cellular respiration
5. ATP
6. Oxygen; Nutrients
7. Building; Synthetic

V. HOMEOSTATIC MECHANISMS MAINTAIN AN APPROPRIATE INTERNAL ENVIRONMENT
1. Homeostasis
2. Stressor
3. Feedback system
4. Negative feedback
5. Negative
6. Positive feedback
7. Positive

VI. THE BODY HAS A BASIC PLAN
1. Mirror; Bilateral
2. Cranium; Vertebral column

A. Directions in the Body Are Relative
1. Anatomical
2. Superior
3. Inferior
4. Closer
5. Cephalic
6. Caudal
7. Anterior; Ventral
8. Posterior; Dorsal
9. Axis
10. Medial
11. Midline
12. Lateral
13. Proximal
14. Distal
15. Superficial
16. Deep

B. The Body Has Three Main Planes
1. Axes
2. Sagittal plane
3. Midsagittal plane
4. Transverse plane
5. Frontal plane

C. We Can Identify Specific Body Regions

1. Axial
2. Appendicular
3. Torso
4. Cephalic
5. Cervical
6. Cranial

D. The Body Has Two Main Cavities

1. Cavities
2. Dorsal; Ventral
3. Cranial; Vertebral
4. Thoracic; Abdominopelvic
5. Diaphragm
6. Pericardial

E. It Is Important to View the Body as a Whole

Figure 1-1: See Figure 1-8B in your textbook.
Figure 1-2: See Figure 1-10 in your textbook.

CHAPTER TEST

1. a
2. b
3. b
4. c
5. c
6. a
7. a
8. a
9. b
10. a
11. b
12. b
13. c
14. c
15. b
16. a
17. c
18. b

CHAPTER 2

STUDY QUESTIONS

I. THE CELL CONTAINS SPECIALIZED ORGANELLES THAT PERFORM SPECIFIC FUNCTIONS

1. Cells
2. Microscope
3. Light
4. Electron
5. Functions
6. Ovum
7. Cytoplasm
8. Amino Acids
9. Organelles
10. Plasma
11. Receptors
12. Nucleus
13. Chromosomes
14. DNA
15. Genome
16. Nucleolus
17. Endoplasmic reticulum
18. Smooth; Rough
19. Ribosomes
20. Proteins
21. Golgi complex
22. Lysosomes
23. Mitochondria
24. Cellular respiration
25. Free radicals
26. Cilia

Figure 2-1: See Figure 2-2 in your textbook.

II. MATERIALS MOVE THROUGH THE PLASMA MEMBRANE

1. Permeable
2. Diffusion
3. Osmosis
4. Filtration
5. Active transport
6. Phagocytosis

III. CELLS DIVIDE BY MITOSIS, FORMING GENETICALLY IDENTICAL CELLS

1. Mitosis
2. Chromosomes
3. Five
4. Interphase
5. Prophase
6. Metaphase
7. Anaphase
8. Telophase
9. Two

IV. TISSUES ARE THE FABRIC OF THE BODY

1. Tissue
2. Epithelial; Connective; Muscle; Nervous (in any order)
3. Histology

A. Epithelial Protects the Body

1. Epithelial
2. Absorb
3. Squamous
4. Cuboidal
5. Columnar
6. Simple; Stratified
7. Pseudostratified
8. Gland
9. Exocrine; Endocrine

10. Thyroid

B. Connective Tissue Joins Body Structures
1. Join together
2. Organ
3. Intercellular; Fibers
4. Collagen; Reticular; Elastic (any order)
5. Fibroblasts; Macrophages
6. Loose
7. Adipose

C. Muscle Tissue Is Specialized to Contract
1. Contract
2. Skeletal
3. Involuntary
4. Smooth

D. Nervous Tissue Controls Muscles and Glands
1. Neurons; Glial
2. Cell body
3. Dendrites; Axon
4. Sensory

V. MEMBRANES COVER OR LINE BODY SURFACES
1. Membranes
2. Mucous
3. Serous
4. Synovial
5. Parietal
6. Visceral

Figure 2-2: See Figure 2-6 in your textbook.

CHAPTER TEST

1. c
2. d
3. b
4. b
5. a
6. c
7. c
8. a
9. d
10. b
11. d
12. d
13. c
14. b
15. a
16. a
17. b
18. c
19. d
20. d
21. c
22. d
23. a
24. b
25. b
26. b

CHAPTER 3

STUDY QUESTIONS

I. THE SKIN FUNCTIONS AS A PROTECTIVE BARRIER
1. Integumentary system
2. Sensory receptors
3. Fluid
4. Vitamin D

II. THE SKIN CONSISTS OF THE EPIDERMIS AND DERMIS
1. Epidermis
2. Dermis
3. Subcutaneous

A. The Epidermis Continuously Replaces Itself
1. Epithelial
2. Outer
3. Deepest
4. Keratin
5. Die

B. The Dermis Provides Strength and Elasticity
1. Connective
2. Collagen
3. Hair follicles; Glands
4. Papillae
5. Temperature
6. Fingerprints

C. The Subcutaneous Layer Attaches the Skin to Underlying Tissues
1. Superficial fascia
2. Muscles
3. Shock
4. Adipose
5. Fat

III. SWEAT GLANDS HELP MAINTAIN BODY TEMPERATURE
1. Sweat glands
2. Body temperature
3. Heat; Increase
4. Evaporation
5. Nitrogen
6. Sweat
7. Armpits; Genital

IV. SEBACEOUS GLANDS LUBRICATE THE HAIR AND SKIN
1. Sebaceous glands
2. Ducts
3. Sebum
4. Pimple
5. Acne

V. HAIR AND NAILS ARE APPENDAGES OF THE SKIN
1. Protective
2. Palms; Soles
3. Shaft
4. Root
5. Follicle
6. Capillaries
7. Keratin
8. Dead
9. Smooth
10. Contract
11. Nails

VI. MELANIN HELPS DETERMINE SKIN COLOR
1. Lowest
2. Melanin
3. Color
4. Carotene
5. Albino

6. Sun
7. Absorbs
8. Darker
9. Ultraviolet
10. Sunburned
11. Cancer

Figure 3-1: See Figure 3-1 in your textbook.

CHAPTER TEST
1. c
2. b
3. d
4. c
5. a
6. b
7. c
8. b
9. b
10. b
11. b
12. a
13. b
14. a
15. a
16. c
17. d
18. d
19. d

SOLUTION TO CROSSWORD PUZZLE FOR CHAPTERS 1, 2, AND 3

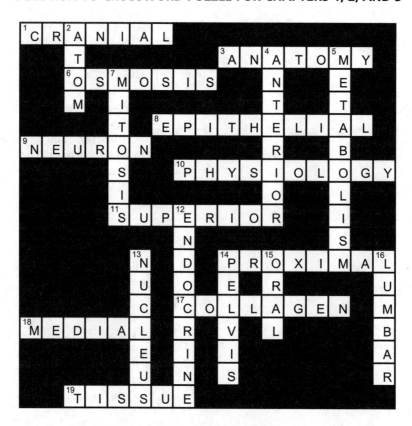

CHAPTER 4

STUDY QUESTIONS

I. THE SKELETAL SYSTEM SUPPORTS AND PROTECTS THE BODY

1. Support; Protect
2. Bones
3. Tendons
4. Ligaments
5. Marrow
6. Interaction

II. A TYPICAL LONG BONE CONSISTS OF A SHAFT WITH FLARED ENDS

1. Diaphysis
2. Epiphysis
3. Metaphysis
4. Epiphyseal
5. Hyaline
6. Periosteum
7. Bone
8. Yellow
9. Endosteum

III. TWO TYPES OF BONE TISSUE ARE COMPACT AND SPONGY BONE

1. Compact; Spongy
2. Dense
3. Spindle; Osteons
4. Osteocytes; Lacunae
5. Haversian canals
6. Canaliculi
7. Epiphyses
8. Bone marrow
9. Red; Yellow

IV. BONE DEVELOPS BY REPLACING EXISTING CONNECTIVE TISSUE

1. Ossification
2. Fetal
3. Endochondral
4. Intramembranous
5. Osteoblasts
6. Hydroxyapatite
7. Lacunae
8. Osteocytes
9. Osteoclasts; Resorption
10. Enzymes
11. Shape
12. Bones
13. Tissue; Marrow

Figure 4-1: See Figure 4-1B in your textbook.

V. THE BONES OF THE SKELETON ARE GROUPED IN TWO DIVISIONS

1. 206
2. Axial
3. Appendicular

Figure 4-2: See Figure 4-2 in your textbook.

VI. THE AXIAL SKELETON CONSISTS OF 80 BONES

1. Parietal
2. Mandible; Temporomandibular
3. Sternum
4. Atlas
5. Ribs

A. The Skull Is the Bony Framework of the Head

1. Cranium; Face
2. Middle
3. Sutures
4. Sagittal suture
5. Frontal
6. Lambdoid suture
7. Fontanelles
8. Anterior; Coronal
9. Soft spots
10. Sinuses
11. Paranasal
12. Sinusitis

B. The Vertebral Column Supports the Body

1. Spine
2. 24
3. Sacrum; Coccyx
4. Cervical; Thoracic; 5; Fused; Coccygeal
5. Intervertebral discs
6. Discs
7. Vertebral foramen

Figure 4-3: See Figure 4-5 in your textbook.
Figure 4-4: See Figure 4-6 in your textbook.
Figure 4-5: See Figure 4-8 in your textbook.

C. The Thoracic Cage Protects the Organs of the Chest

1. Rib
2. Pectoral
3. Sternum; Thoracic; 12

Figure 4-6: See Figure 4-9A in your textbook.
Figure 4-7: See Figure 4-10A, C, D, and E in your textbook.

VII. THE APPENDICULAR SKELETON CONSISTS OF 126 BONES

1. Appendicular; Pectoral; Pelvic
2. Femur
3. Patella
4. Humerus
5. Metacarpals

A. The Pectoral Girdle Attaches the Upper Extremities (Limbs) to the Axial Skeleton
1. Clavicle
2. Sternum
3. Glenoid
4. Spine

B. The Bones of the Upper Extremity (Limb) Are Located in the Arm, Forearm, Wrist, and Hand
1. 30
2. Humerus
3. Radius; Ulna
4. Carpal
5. Metacarpal
6. Phalanges
Figure 4-8: See Figure 4-11 in your textbook.

C. The Pelvic Girdle Supports the Lower Limbs
1. Pelvic
2. Coxal
3. Sacrum; Coccyx
4. Ilium
5. Ischium
6. Pubis
7. Symphysis
Figure 4-9: See Figure 4-12A in your textbook.

D. Bones of the Lower Extremity (Limb) Are Located in the Thigh, Knee, Leg, Ankle, and Foot
1. 30
2. Femur
3. Patella
4. Fibula; Tibia
5. Tarsal
6. Metatarsal
7. Phalanges
Figure 4-10: See Figure 4-13 in your textbook.

VIII. JOINTS ARE JUNCTIONS BETWEEN BONES
1. Articulation
2. Ball-and-socket
3. Hinge
4. Pivot

A. Joints Can Be Classified According to the Degree of Movement They Permit
1. Three
2. Synarthroses; Fibrous
3. Skull
4. Amphiarthroses; Cartilage
5. Intervertebral
6. Diarthroses
7. Synovial

B. A Diarthrosis Is Surrounded by a Joint Capsule
1. Hyaline
2. Joint
3. Ligaments
4. Synovial
5. Bursae
6. Bursitis

CHAPTER TEST
1. d
2. c
3. b
4. c
5. a
6. b
7. c
8. d
9. d
10. a
11. d
12. d
13. a
14. b
15. c
16. c
17. d
18. b
19. d
20. a
21. a
22. a
23. c
24. b
Figure 4-11: See Figure 4-3 in your textbook.

CHAPTER 5

STUDY QUESTIONS

INTRODUCTION
1. Muscles
2. Skeletal; Smooth; Cardiac (in any order)
3. Voluntary

I. SKELETAL MUSCLE IS COMPOSED OF HUNDREDS OF MUSCLE FIBERS
1. Fibers
2. Epimysium
3. Fascicles
4. Perimysium
5. Endomysium
6. Tendons

II. MUSCLE FIBERS ARE SPECIALIZED FOR CONTRACTION
1. Mitochondria
2. Transverse
3. Myofibrils
4. Filaments
5. Myosin
6. Actin
7. Contractile
8. Sarcomeres

A. Contraction Occurs When Actin and Myosin Filaments Slide Past Each Other
1. Bones
2. Fibers
3. Motor
4. Impulses
5. Neuromuscular
6. Acetylcholine
7. Synaptic
8. Action
9. Acetylcholinesterase
10. Calcium
11. Bridges

B. Muscle Contraction Requires Energy
1. ATP
2. Creatine phosphate
3. Fuel
4. Glucose
5. Muscle fatigue
6. Lactic acid
7. Oxygen debt

C. Muscle Tone Is a State of Partial Contraction
1. Muscle tone
2. Unconscious
3. Posture
4. Motor nerve

D. Two Types of Muscle Contraction Are Isotonic and Isometric
1. Isotonic
2. Isometric

III. MUSCLES WORK ANTAGONISTICALLY TO ONE ANOTHER
1. Tendons
2. Articulates
3. Origin
4. Insertion
5. Agonist
6. Antagonist
7. Synergists
8. Fixators

IV. WE CAN STUDY MUSCLES IN FUNCTIONAL GROUPS
1. Masseter
2. Trapezius
3. Rectus abdominis
4. Diaphragm
5. Pectoralis
6. Biceps brachii
7. Gluteus maximus
8. Gastrocnemius

Figure 5-1: See Figure 5-7 in your textbook.
Figure 5-2: See Figure 5-8 in your textbook.

CHAPTER TEST
1. d
2. a
3. b
4. c
5. d
6. b
7. b
8. c
9. c
10. a
11. b
12. a
13. d
14. c
15. a
16. b
17. a
18. b
19. c
20. b
21. a

SOLUTION TO CROSSWORD PUZZLE FOR CHAPTERS 4 AND 5

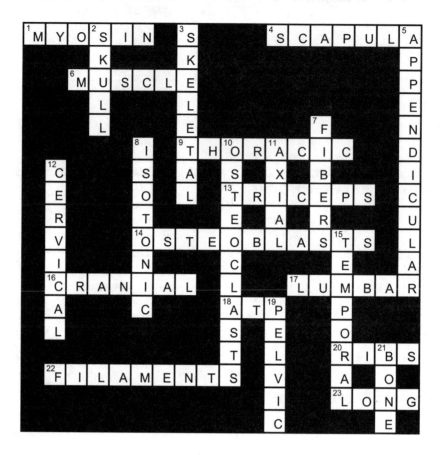

CHAPTER 6

STUDY QUESTIONS

I. THE NERVOUS SYSTEM HAS TWO MAIN DIVISIONS
1. Central; Peripheral
2. Brain
3. Sense
4. Cranial; Spinal
5. Somatic; Autonomic
6. Afferent
7. Efferent

II. NEURONS AND GLIAL CELLS ARE THE CELLS OF THE NERVOUS SYSTEM
1. Glial
2. Neurons
3. Fibers
4. Dendrites
5. Axon
6. Neurotransmitters
7. Myelin; Cellular
8. Sheath
9. Impulses

Figure 6-1: See Figure 6-2A in your textbook.

III. BUNDLES OF AXONS MAKE UP NERVES
1. Nerve
2. Axons; Myelin
3. Ganglion
4. Tracts
5. Nuclei

IV. APPROPRIATE RESPONSES DEPEND ON NEURAL SIGNALING
1. Correct order is: 3; 1; 4; 2; 5
   Reception
   Transmission (to the CNS)
   Integration
   Transmission (to the muscles)
   Actual response
2. Interneurons
3. Dendrites
4. Synapse
5. Synaptic
6. Neurotransmitters

V. NEURONS USE ELECTRICAL SIGNALS TO TRANSMIT INFORMATION
1. Plasma
2. Polarized
3. Potential

A. The Neuron Has a Resting Potential
1. Resting
2. millivolts
3. Passive ion
4. Sodium-Potassium
5. Sodium; Potassium

B. An Action Potential Is a Wave of Depolarization
1. Impulses
2. Permeability
3. Hyperpolarization
4. Voltage-activated
5. Action potential
6. Repolarization
7. Unmyelinated
8. Ranvier

VI. NEURONS SIGNAL OTHER CELLS ACROSS SYNAPSES
1. Synapse
2. Presynaptic
3. Postsynaptic
4. Synaptic cleft

A. Neurons Use Neurotransmitters to Signal Other Cells
1. Neurotransmitters
2. Chemical
3. Neuromodulators
4. Cholinergic
5. Adrenergic
6. Catecholamines
7. Amino
8. Endorphins; Enkephalins
9. Nitric oxide

B. Neurotransmitters Bind With Receptors on Postsynaptic Neurons
1. Synaptic vesicles
2. Receptors
3. Ion
4. Reuptake
5. Dopamine

C. Neurotransmitter Receptors Can Send Excitatory or Inhibitory Signals
1. Excitatory; Inhibitory
2. Excitatory postsynaptic potential (EPSP)
3. Inhibitory postsynaptic potential (IPSP)
4. Summation

VII. NEURAL IMPULSES MUST BE INTEGRATED
1. Neural integration
2. Cancel
3. Graded
4. Action potential
5. CNS

VIII. THE HUMAN BRAIN IS THE MOST COMPLEX MECHANISM KNOWN
1. Neural
2. Oxygen; Glucose
3. Stroke
4. Cerebrovascular
5. Ventricles

A. The Medulla Contains Vital Centers
1. Oblongata
2. Spinal cord
3. Reticular formation
4. Cerebrum
5. Cardiac
6. Vasomotor
7. Respiratory
8. Medulla

B. The Pons Is a Bridge to Other Parts of the Brain
1. Pons
2. Medulla
3. Cerebellum
4. Brain
5. Nerve
6. Respiration

C. The Midbrain Contains Centers for Visual and Auditory Reflexes
1. Midbrain
2. Pons
3. Cerebral aqueduct
4. Neurons
5. Visual; Auditory

D. The Diencephalon Includes the Thalamus and the Hypothalamus
1. Diencephalon
2. Thalamus
3. Nuclei
4. Motor
5. Hypothalamus
6. Autonomic
7. Endocrine
8. Motivational
9. Circadian
10. Suprachiasmatic

E. The Cerebellum Is Responsible for Coordination of Movement
1. Cerebellum
2. Movements
3. Muscle
4. Vestibular
5. Motor

6. Language

F. The Cerebrum Is the Largest Part of the Brain
1. Cerebrum
2. Sensory; Motor; Association (any order)
3. Movement
4. Intellectual
5. Transverse
6. Corpus callosum
7. Frontal
8. Parietal
9. Primary visual area
10. Temporal

G. The Limbic System Affects Emotional Aspects of Behavior
1. Limbic
2. Motivation
3. Hippocampus; Amygdala
4. Memories
5. Emotional

Figure 6-2: See Figure 6-8 in your textbook.

H. Learning Involves Many Areas of the Brain
1. Learning
2. Memory
3. Synaptic plasticity

IX. THE SPINAL CORD TRANSMITS INFORMATION TO AND FROM THE BRAIN
1. Spinal
2. Vertebral
3. Fissures
4. Ascending
5. Descending

Figure 6-3: See Figure 6-12A in your textbook.

X. THE CENTRAL NERVOUS SYSTEM IS WELL-PROTECTED

A. The Meninges Are Connective Tissue Coverings
1. Meninges
2. Dura mater
3. Sinuses
4. Arachnoid
5. Pia mater
6. Meningitis
7. Encephalitis

B. The Cerebrospinal Fluid Cushions the CNS
1. Cerebrospinal
2. Choroid plexuses
3. Brain
4. Hydrocephalus
5. Lumbar

XI. A REFLEX ACTION IS A SIMPLE NEURAL RESPONSE
1. Reflex
2. Regulation
3. Inhibit

Figure 6-4: See Figure 6-13 in your textbook.

CHAPTER TEST
1. b
2. c
3. b
4. a
5. a
6. b
7. c
8. d
9. d
10. d
11. d
12. d

CHAPTER 7

STUDY QUESTIONS

INTRODUCTION
1. Sensory
2. Somatic
3. Autonomic

I. THE SOMATIC DIVISION RESPONDS TO CHANGES IN THE OUTSIDE WORLD
1. Somatic
2. Cranial; Spinal

A. Cranial Nerves Link the Brain With Sensory Receptors and Muscles
1. Cranial
2. Sensory
3. CNS
4. Afferent; Efferent

B. Spinal Nerves Link the Spinal Cord With Various Structures
1. Spinal
2. Vertebral column
3. Eight
4. Thoracic
5. Lumbar
6. Five
7. Coccygeal
8. Dorsal
9. Ganglion
10. Ventral

1. ***Each Spinal Nerve Divides Into Branches and the Ventral Branches Form Plexuses***
1. Branches
2. Dorsal
3. Ventral
4. Plexuses
5. Innervate
6. Cervical; Brachial; Lumbar; Sacral
7. Femoral
8. Sciatic
Figure 7-1: See Figure 7-3 in your textbook.

II. THE AUTONOMIC DIVISION MAINTAINS INTERNAL BALANCE
1. Autonomic
2. Sympathetic; Parasympathetic
3. Efferent

A. The Sympathetic System Mobilizes Energy
1. Action
2. Sympathetic
3. Neurons
4. Paravertebral
5. Collateral
6. Preganglionic
7. Postganglionic
8. Acetylcholine; Cholinergic
9. Norepinephrine; Adrenergic

B. The Parasympathetic System Conserves and Restores Energy
1. Active
2. Conserving
3. Brain
4. Vagus
5. Terminal ganglia
6. Pelvic
7. Parasympathetic
8. Acetylcholine

CHAPTER TEST
1. a
2. c
3. b
4. d
5. d
6. c
7. b
8. a
9. a
10. b
11. b
12. b

CHAPTER 8

STUDY QUESTIONS

INTRODUCTION
1. Stimulus
2. Sensory
3. Eyes; Ears; Nose; Taste buds (any order)
4. Receptors

I. SENSORY RECEPTORS PRODUCE RECEPTOR POTENTIALS
1. Stimulus
2. Transduction
3. Receptor potential
4. Depolarized
5. CNS

II. WE CAN CLASSIFY SENSORY RECEPTORS ACCORDING TO THE TYPE OF ENERGY THEY TRANSDUCE
1. Mechanoreceptors
2. Chemoreceptors
3. Photoreceptors
4. Thermoreceptors

III. THE EYE CONTAINS PHOTORECEPTORS
1. Orbit
2. Fat
3. Eyelashes; Eyelids
4. Reflex
5. Blinking
6. Lacrimal glands
7. Lacrimal duct
8. Extrinsic
9. Cornea; Choroid; Retina
10. Sclera
11. Conjunctiva
12. Iris
13. Light
14. Pupil
15. Lens
16. Aqueous humor
17. Vitreous humor
18. Suspensory ligament

A. The Eye Can Be Compared to a Camera
1. Retina
2. Accommodation
3. Ciliary
4. Relaxes; Ovoid
5. Presbyopia

B. The Retina Contains Light-Sensitive Rods and Cones
1. Photoreceptors
2. Cones
3. Rods
4. Fovea
5. Bipolar; Ganglion
6. Optic
7. Optic disc
8. Rhodopsin

C. The Optic Nerve Transmits Signals to the Brain
1. Optic nerves
2. Optic chiasm
3. Lateral geniculate
4. Primary visual cortex
5. Trigeminal nerve
6. Cerebrum

Figure 8-1: See Figure 8-1 in your textbook.

IV. THE EAR FUNCTIONS IN HEARING AND EQUILIBRIUM
1. Outer
2. Middle
3. Sensory; Equilibrium

A. The Outer Ear Conducts Sound Waves to the Middle Ear
1. Pinna
2. External auditory meatus
3. Ceruminous
4. Cerumen
5. Tympanic membrane

B. The Middle Ear Amplifies Sound Waves
1. Middle ear; Ossicles
2. Eustachian
3. Malleus; Incus; Stapes
4. Oval window
5. Tympanic membrane
6. Vibrations

C. The Inner Ear Contains Mechanoreceptors
1. Mechanoreceptors
2. Equilibrium
3. Labyrinth
4. Vestibule; Cochlea; Semicircular canals
5. Perilymph
6. Membranous
7. Endolymph
8. Vibrations

1. The Cochlea Contains the Receptors for Hearing
1. Cochlea
2. Organ of Corti

3. Cochlear nerve
4. Vestibular; Tympanic; Perilymph
5. Cochlear
6. Hair
7. Stereocilia
8. Basilar

2. Sounds Vary in Pitch, Loudness, and Quality
1. Pitch
2. Low-frequency
3. High-frequency
4. Hair
5. Amplitude
6. Cochlear
7. Deafness
8. High-intensity

D. The Vestibule and Semicircular Canals Help Maintain Equilibrium
1. Vestibule; Semicircular
2. Saccule; Utricle
3. Otoliths
4. Cupula
5. Angular acceleration
6. Crista
7. Endolymph
8. Vestibular; Vestibulocochlear

Figure 8-2: See Figure 8-5 in your textbook.

V. SMELL IS SENSED BY CHEMORECEPTORS IN THE NASAL CAVITY
1. Olfactory
2. Olfactory nerve; Temporal
3. Odors; Scents

VI. TASTE BUDS DETECT DISSOLVED FOOD MOLECULES
1. Gustation; Taste buds
2. Papillae
3. Taste receptors
4. Regenerated
5. Sweet; Sour; Salty; Bitter (any order)
6. Tip
7. Sides; Posterior
8. Smell; Taste

VII. THE GENERAL SENSES ARE WIDESPREAD THROUGHOUT THE BODY
1. Touch, Pressure, Vibration, Pain (any order); Temperature; Muscle

A. Tactile Receptors Are Located in the Skin
1. Mechanoreceptors
2. Touch; Pressure; Pain (any order)
3. Tactile

B. Temperature Receptors Are Nerve Endings

1. Thermoreceptors
2. Lips; Mouth
3. Skin; Temperature
4. Hypothalamus; Homeostatic

C. Pain Sensation Is a Protective Mechanism

1. Pain
2. Nociceptors
3. Thermal
4. Mechanical
5. Glutamate; Substance P
6. Analgesia
7. Beta-endorphins; Enkephalins
8. Phantom pain
9. Referred
10. Acupuncture

D. Proprioceptors Inform Us of Our Position

1. Proprioceptors
2. Muscle spindles
3. Golgi tendon organs
4. Ligaments
5. Vestibule; Semicircular; Equilibrium

CHAPTER TEST

1. d
2. a
3. a
4. a
5. b
6. b
7. d
8. a
9. d
10. c
11. d
12. a
13. b
14. c
15. b
16. c
17. b
18. a
19. a
20. b.
21. c
22. c
23. b
24. a
25. b

CHAPTER 9

STUDY QUESTIONS

INTRODUCTION

1. Growth, Reproduction; Cells; Fluid; Metabolic
2. Endocrinology
3. Endocrine; Hormones
4. Exocrine
5. Target
6. Homeostasis

I. MANY TISSUES SECRETE HORMONES OR HORMONE-LIKE SUBSTANCES

1. Neuroendocrine
2. Neurohormones
3. Blood
4. Prostaglandins
5. Hormones

II. HORMONES COMBINE WITH SPECIFIC RECEPTORS ON OR IN TARGET CELLS

1. Target
2. Receptors
3. First messenger

A. Many Hormones Act Through Second Messengers and Steroid Hormones Activate Genes

1. Plasma
2. Second messenger
3. Calcium
4. Calmodulin
5. Cyclic AMP
6. Steroid

III. HORMONE SECRETION IS REGULATED BY NEGATIVE FEEDBACK MECHANISMS

1. Homeostasis
2. Negative feedback
3. Endocrine gland
4. Parathyroid
5. Hyposecretion
6. Hypersecretion

IV. THE HYPOTHALAMUS REGULATES THE PITUITARY GLAND

1. Hypothalamus
2. Endocrine
3. Pituitary gland
4. Releasing; inhibiting
5. Anterior; posterior

A. The Posterior Lobe Releases Two Hormones Produced by the Hypothalamus
1. Posterior lobe
2. Oxytocin
3. Labor
4. Antidiuretic hormone (ADH)
5. Inhibits
6. Diabetes insipidus

B. The Anterior Lobe Regulates Growth and Other Endocrine Glands
1. Anterior lobe
2. Tropic
3. Releasing; Inhibiting
4. Portal
5. Prolactin
6. Thyroid
7. Adrenal cortex
8. Gonadotropic

1. Growth Hormone Stimulates Protein Synthesis
1. Growth hormone
2. Somatomedins; Insulin-like growth factors
3. Hypothalamus; Pituitary
4. Increases
5. Pulses
6. Psychosocial dwarfism
7. Sex

V. THYROID HORMONES INCREASE METABOLIC RATE
1. Thyroid gland
2. Thyroid hormones
3. Thyroxine
4. T_3
5. Negative feedback system
6. Thyroid stimulating hormone
7. Hypothyroidism
8. Goiter
9. Hyposecretion; Hypersecretion

VI. PARATHYROID GLANDS REGULATE CALCIUM CONCENTRATION
1. Parathyroid glands
2. Parathyroid hormones
3. Increases
4. Vitamin D
5. Calcium
6. Calcitonin

VII. THE ISLETS OF LANGERHANS REGULATE GLUCOSE CONCENTRATION
1. Posterior
2. Exocrine; Endocrine
3. Digestive
4. Islets of Langerhans

5. Beta cells
6. Alpha
7. Insulin
8. Glucose
9. Glucagon
10. Opposite
11. Antagonistically

A. In Diabetes Mellitus, Glucose Accumulates in the Blood
1. Diabetes mellitus
2. Type 1
3. Insulin
4. Type 2
5. Insulin resistance
6. Urine

VIII. THE ADRENAL GLANDS FUNCTION IN METABOLISM AND STRESS
1. Adrenal glands
2. Adrenal medulla; Adrenal cortex
3. Metabolism; Stress

A. The Adrenal Medulla Secretes Epinephrine and Norepinephrine
1. Adrenal medulla
2. Epinephrine; Norepinephrine
3. Neurotransmitter
4. Emergency
5. Metabolic
6. Dilate

B. The Adrenal Cortex Secretes Steroid Hormones
1. Adrenal cortex
2. Glucocorticoids
3. Cortisol
4. Glucose
5. Mineralocorticoids
6. Aldosterone
7. Sodium; Potassium
8. Androgen; Estrogen
9. Corticotropin releasing factor
10. Adrenocorticotropic hormone

C. Stress Threatens Homeostasis
1. Homeostasis
2. Stressors
3. Sympathetic; Adrenal
4. Epinephrine; Norepinephrine
5. Hormones

Figure 9-1: See Figure 9-4 in your textbook.

CHAPTER TEST
1. c
2. d
3. a

4.	b	12.	b
5.	c	13.	d
6.	d	14.	c
7.	a	15.	a
8.	a	16.	b
9.	b	17.	b
10.	c	18.	d
11.	a	19.	d

SOLUTION TO CROSSWORD PUZZLE FOR CHAPTERS 6, 7, 8, AND 9

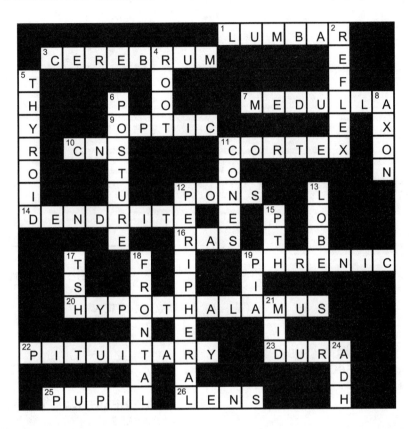

CHAPTER 10

STUDY QUESTIONS

INTRODUCTION
1. Circulatory
2. Cardiovascular; Lymphatic
3. Heart
4. Blood
5. Fluid; Disease
6. Platelets; Plasma

I. PLASMA IS THE FLUID COMPONENT OF BLOOD
1. Water
2. Interstitial fluid; Intracellular fluid
3. Plasma proteins

4. Liver
5. Albumins; Globulins; Fibrinogen (any order)
6. Acid-base; pH
7. Alpha globulins
8. Prothrombin
9. Beta
10. Gamma
11. Serum

II. RED BLOOD CELLS TRANSPORT OXYGEN
1. Red blood cells
2. Hemoglobin
3. Biconcave; Oxygen
4. Nucleus
5. Oxyhemoglobin
6. Marrow
7. Stem cells
8. Erythropoietin

9. Kidneys
10. Anemia
11. Iron deficiency

III. WHITE BLOOD CELLS DEFEND THE BODY AGAINST DISEASE
1. Leukocytes
2. Tissues
3. Phagocytosis
4. Phagocytes
5. Granular
6. Neutrophils; Basophils; Eosinophils (any order)
7. Bacteria
8. Enzymes
9. Lysosomes
10. Allergic reactions; Parasitic
11. Histamine
12. Heparin
13. Lymphocytes; Monocytes
14. Antibodies; Attack
15. Macrophages

IV. PLATELETS FUNCTION IN BLOOD CLOTTING
1. Thrombocytes
2. Prevent
3. Platelet plug
4. Clotting factors; Prothrombin activator
5. Thrombin
6. Liver; Vitamin K
7. Fibrinogen
8. Fibrin
9. Serum

V. SUCCESSFUL BLOOD TRANSFUSIONS DEPEND ON BLOOD GROUPS
1. Transfusions; Donors; Recipients
2. Centrifuge
3. Plasma
4. Whole
5. Transfusion reaction
6. Antibodies; Agglutinate
7. Hemolysis

A. The ABO Blood Groups Are Based on Antigens A and B
1. Antigens
2. Universal donors
3. Antibodies
4. Anti-B
5. Anti-A
6. Type O
7. Repeated
8. Universal recipients

B. The Rh System Consists of Several Rh Antigens
1. Rh antigens
2. Rh factor

3. Antigen D
4. Rh positive; Red blood cells
5. Rh negative
6. Exposed
7. Rh incompatibility
8. Hemolytic anemia

CHAPTER TEST
1. b
2. d
3. d
4. d
5. a
6. a
7. a
8. c
9. d
10. b
11. c
12. a
13. c
14. d
15. b

CHAPTER 11

STUDY QUESTIONS

INTRODUCTION
1. Organ
2. Blood
3. Thorax
4. Midline

I. THE HEART WALL CONSISTS OF THREE LAYERS
1. Heart; Blood; Lymph
2. Endocardium; Myocardium; Pericardium (Epicardium)
3. Endothelial
4. Cardiac
5. Epicardium; Visceral
6. Pericardial cavity
7. Parietal

II. THE HEART HAS FOUR CHAMBERS
1. Heart
2. Septum
3. Atria
4. Ventricles
5. Pulmonary
6. Interatrial
7. Interventricular
8. Auricle
Figure 11-1: See Figure 11-1 in your textbook.

III. VALVES PREVENT BACKFLOW OF BLOOD
1. Atrioventricular
2. Cusps
3. Tricuspid
4. Bicuspid
5. Mitral
6. Mitral stenosis
7. Semilunar
8. Aortic
9. Pulmonary

IV. THE HEART HAS ITS OWN BLOOD VESSELS
1. Oxygen
2. Cardiac
3. Coronary
4. Coronary arteries
5. Coronary veins
6. Coronary sinus; Right atrium

V. THE CONDUCTION SYSTEM CONSISTS OF SPECIALIZED CARDIAC MUSCLES
1. Conduction
2. Sinoatrial
3. Atrioventricular
4. Bundle
5. Myocardium
6. Intercalated

VI. THE CARDIAC CYCLE INCLUDES CONTRACTION AND RELAXATION PHASES
1. Cardiac cycle
2. Systole
3. Diastole
4. Atria
5. Ventricles
6. Semilunar
7. Veins
8. Arteries
9. Electrocardiogram

VII. CLOSURE OF THE VALVES CAUSES THE HEART SOUNDS
1. Stethoscope; Lub-dup
2. Ventricular
3. Diastole
4. Heart murmurs
5. Blood; Hissing
6. Valve

VIII. CARDIAC OUTPUT VARIES WITH THE BODY'S NEEDS
1. Cardiac output
2. Stroke volume
3. Ventricle; Cardiac
4. Heart rate
5. Venous
6. Starling's; Heart
7. Norepinephrine

IX. THE HEART IS REGULATED BY THE NERVOUS AND ENDOCRINE SYSTEMS
1. Blood pressure
2. Cardiac centers
3. Autonomic; SA
4. Acetylcholine
5. Norepinephrine
6. Beta-adrenergic
7. Tachycardia
8. Bradycardia
9. Decreases

Figure 11-2: See Figure 11-2 in your textbook.

CHAPTER TEST
1. c
2. a
3. c
4. a
5. b
6. b
7. a
8. c
9. a
10. d
11. c
12. b
13. c
14. a
15. b
16. b
17. a
18. c
19. b
20. a
21. d
22. c
23. a
24. b
25. c
26. d

CHAPTER 12

STUDY QUESTIONS

INTRODUCTION
1. Blood vessels
2. Smaller
3. Interstitial; Tissue
4. Nourishes

I. THREE MAIN TYPES OF BLOOD VESSELS ARE ARTERIES, CAPILLARIES, AND VEINS
1. Arteries
2. Pulmonary
3. Arterioles

4. Capillaries
5. Exchanged
6. Veins
7. Venules
8. Oxygen
9. Tunics
10. Endothelium
11. Connective
12. Collagen
13. Valves; Heart
14. Metarterioles
15. Sinusoids
16. Macrophages

Figure 12-1: See Figure 12-1 in your textbook.

II. BLOOD CIRCULATES THROUGH TWO CIRCUITS

1. Pulmonary
2. Systemic
3. Ventricle
4. Right
5. Carbon dioxide; Oxygen

A. The Pulmonary Circulation Carries Blood To and From the Lungs

1. Atrium
2. Pulmonary
3. Pulmonary veins; Left atrium
4. 3; 2; 1; 4; 6; 5

B. The Systemic Circulation Carries Blood to the Tissues

1. The Aorta Has Four Main Regions

1. Ascending
2. Aortic arch
3. Thoracic
4. Abdominal
5. Descending aorta

2. The Superior and Inferior Venae Cavae Return Blood to the Heart

1. Carbon dioxide
2. Capillaries; Veins
3. Superior vena cava
4. Inferior vena cava
5. Right atrium

3. Four Arteries Supply the Brain

1. Arteries
2. Internal carotid
3. Vertebral; Basilar
4. Circle of Willis
5. Anastomosis
6. Venous sinuses
7. Internal jugular
8. Brachiocephalic; Superior; Heart

9. 1; 9; 2; 4; 3; 6; 5; 8; 7

Figure 12-2: See Figure 12-3 in your textbook.

4. The Liver Has an Unusual Circulation

1. Portal
2. Hepatic
3. Mesenteric
4. Superior mesenteric
5. Liver; Homeostatic
6. Toxic

III. SEVERAL FACTORS INFLUENCE BLOOD FLOW

A. The Alternate Expansion and Recoil of an Artery Is Its Pulse

1. Pumps blood
2. Arterial
3. Systole
4. Diastole
5. Artery
6. Radial; Carotid artery
7. Pulse

B. Blood Pressure Depends on Blood Flow and Resistance to Blood Flow

1. Blood pressure
2. Flow; Resistance
3. Blood
4. Volume
5. Decreases
6. Peripheral resistance
7. Viscosity
8. Diameter

C. Pressure Changes as Blood Flows Through the Systemic Circulation

1. Resistance
2. Arterioles
3. Blood pressure
4. Heart
5. Blood flow
6. Veins
7. Blood
8. Baroreceptors; Constrict
9. Valves

D. Blood Pressure Is Expressed as Systolic Pressure Over Diastolic Pressure

1. Systole; Diastole
2. Blood pressure
3. Normal
4. Numerator; Denominator
5. Sphygmomanometer; Stethoscope
6. Diastolic; Hypertension
7. Vascular resistance
8. Left ventricle

E. Blood Pressure Must Be Carefully Regulated

1. Homeostatic
2. Vasoconstriction
3. Baroreceptors
4. Vasodilation
5. Renin
6. Angiotensinogen; Angiotensin II
7. Aldosterone
8. Blood volume; Blood pressure

IV. THE LYMPHATIC SYSTEM IS A SUBSYSTEM OF THE CIRCULATORY SYSTEM

1. Lymphatic
2. Tissue (Interstitial)
3. Lymphocytes
4. Lymph nodules; Lymph nodes
5. Drainage
6. Blood
7. Lymphatics
8. Thoracic
9. Lymphatic duct

A. Lymph Nodes Filter Lymph

1. Lymph nodes
2. Filter
3. Axillary
4. Macrophages
5. Infection
6. Bacteria

B. Tonsils Filter Tissue Fluid

1. Tonsils
2. Filter
3. Lingual
4. Pharyngeal
5. Adenoids
6. Palatine tonsils
7. Tonsillectomy

C. The Spleen Filters Blood

1. Spleen
2. Blood
3. Filter
4. Bacteria
5. Macrophages
6. Platelets
7. Hemorrhage
8. Splenectomy
9. Bone marrow; Liver

D. The Thymus Gland Plays a Role in Immune Function

1. Thymus gland
2. Puberty
3. Immune
4. Hormones; Lymphocyte

Figure 12-3: See Figure 12-4 in your textbook.
Figure 12-4: See Figure 12-5 in your textbook.

CHAPTER TEST

1. b
2. b
3. d
4. a
5. b
6. c
7. d
8. b
9. a
10. d
11. b
12. d
13. a
14. c
15. c
16. b
17. d
18. a
19. d
20. b
21. b
22. a

CHAPTER 13

STUDY QUESTIONS

INTRODUCTION

1. Pathogens
2. Immunology
3. Immune response
4. Cell signaling
5. Messenger

I. IMMUNE RESPONSES CAN BE NONSPECIFIC OR SPECIFIC

1. Nonspecific immune responses
2. Pathogens
3. Specific immune responses
4. Antigen
5. Antibodies

II. NONSPECIFIC IMMUNE RESPONSES ARE RAPID

1. Nonspecific
2. Barriers
3. Immune
4. Proteins; Inflammation

A. Mechanical and Chemical Barriers Prevent Entry of Most Pathogens

1. Pathogens
2. Skin; Mucous

3. Bacteria
4. Sweat
5. Nose; Respiratory
6. Acids; Enzymes

B. Several Types of Proteins Destroy Pathogens

1. Cytokines Are Important Signaling Molecules

1. Cytokines
2. Interferons
3. Machinery
4. Antiviral
5. Infecting
6. Interleukins
7. Lymphocytes

2. Complement Leads to Pathogen Destruction

1. Complement
2. Antigen
3. Pathogens
4. Destroy
5. Cell wall; Phagocytosis

C. Phagocytes and Natural Killer Cells Destroy Pathogens

1. Phagocytes
2. Phagocytosis
3. Bacterium
4. Neutrophils
5. Macrophages
6. Natural killer
7. Target

D. Inflammation Is a Protective Response

1. Inflammation
2. Edema; Heat; Redness; Pain (any order)
3. Plasma; Mast
4. Histamine; Serotonin
5. Phagocytosis
6. Interstitial; Swelling
7. Fever

III. SPECIFIC DEFENSE MECHANISMS INCLUDE CELL-MEDIATED AND ANTIBODY-MEDIATED IMMUNITY

1. Specific
2. Lymphatic
3. Cell-mediated; Antibody-mediated

A. Many Types of Cells Participate in Specific Immune Responses

1. Lymphocytes
2. Neutrophils; Macrophages; Dendritic (any order)

1. Macrophages and Dendritic Cells Present Antigens

1. Dendritic
2. Interferons; Bacteria
3. Lysosomal
4. Digestive; Urinary; Respiratory; Vaginal (any order)
5. Macrophages
6. Antigen-presenting

2. Lymphocytes Are the Principal Warriors in Specific Immune Responses

1. T; B; Natural killer
2. Virally; Tumor
3. Antibody-mediated; Plasma
4. Cell-mediated
5. Pathogens; Mutation
6. Bone marrow
7. Stem cells
8. Lymph; Thymus
9. Immunological

B. T Cells Are Responsible for Cell-Mediated Immunity

1. T
2. Antigen
3. Cytotoxic T cells
4. Cytokines; Enzymes
5. Helper
6. Suppress
7. Mitosis
8. Memory

C. B Cells Are Responsible for Antibody-Mediated Immunity

1. B
2. Receptor; Antigen
3. Antigen-presenting
4. Helper
5. Plasma; Lymph
6. Memory
7. Antibodies
8. IgG
9. Pathogen
10. Antigen-antibody
11. Deactivate
12. Phagocytes
13. Complement

D. Long-Term Immunity Depends on Memory Cells

1. Immunity
2. Primary response
3. T; Antibodies
4. Nonlymphatic
5. Secondary response
6. Killer
7. Memory

E. Active Immunity Can Be Induced by Immunization

1. Active immunity
2. Immunization; Vaccine
3. Antigens; Memory

F. Passive Immunity Is Borrowed Immunity

1. Passive
2. Effects
3. Antibodies
4. Milk
5. Immunity; Pathogens
6. Immune response; Memory

IV. IMMUNE RESPONSES ARE SOMETIMES INADEQUATE OR HARMFUL

1. Immune
2. Acquired immunodeficiency syndrome; Helper
3. Immune function
4. Antigens; Cancer
5. Antibodies
6. Autoimmune
7. Rejection

CHAPTER TEST

1. a
2. d
3. c
4. b
5. d
6. d
7. c
8. d
9. a
10. c
11. c
12. b
13. d
14. d
15. a
16. a
17. b
18. b
19. d

SOLUTION TO CROSSWORD PUZZLE FOR CHAPTERS 10, 11, 12, AND 13

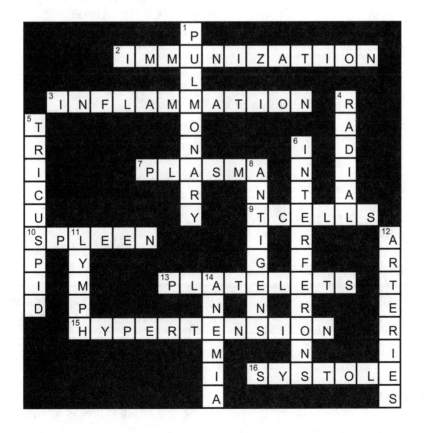

CHAPTER 14

STUDY QUESTIONS

INTRODUCTION
1. Respiration
2. Oxygen; Carbon dioxide
3. Cellular respiration
4. Waste product

I. THE RESPIRATORY SYSTEM CONSISTS OF THE AIRWAY AND LUNGS
1. Respiratory system
2. Nostrils (nares)
3. Larynx
4. Trachea
5. Bronchus
6. Bronchioles; Alveoli
7. Oxygen
8. Lung
9. 3; 2; 5; 1; 4; 8; 7; 6

A. The Nasal Cavities Are Lined With a Mucous Membrane
1. Nares
2. Hairs
3. Nasal septum
4. Mucous
5. Conchae
6. Moistened; Filtered
7. Receptors
8. Throat
9. Sinuses

B. The Pharynx Is Divided Into Three Regions
1. Pharynx
2. Nasopharynx
3. Oropharynx
4. Mouth
5. Laryngopharynx; Larynx
6. Esophagus

C. The Larynx Contains the Vocal Cords
1. Larynx
2. Glottis
3. Adam's apple
4. Laryngitis
5. Vocal cords
6. Lungs
7. Epiglottis
8. Cough

D. The Trachea Is Supported by Rings of Cartilage
1. Trachea
2. Larynx
3. Cartilage

4. Mucous
5. Pharynx
6. Lungs

E. The Bronchi Enter the Lungs
1. Bronchi
2. Bronchioles
3. Bronchial tree
4. Lung

F. Gas Exchange Occurs Through the Alveoli of the Lungs
1. Alveoli
2. Alveolus; Breathing
3. Capillaries
4. Pulmonary surfactant

G. The Lungs Provide a Large Surface Area for Gas Exchange
1. Lungs
2. Mediastinum
3. Lobes
4. Hilus
5. Pleural; Thoracic
6. Visceral; Parietal
7. Pleural cavity
8. Diaphragm

II. VENTILATION MOVES AIR INTO AND OUT OF THE LUNGS
1. Pulmonary
2. Breathing
3. Inspiration
4. Expiration
5. Intercostal
6. Diaphragm
7. Collapsed lung

III. GAS EXCHANGE OCCURS BY DIFFUSION
1. Breathing
2. Circulatory
3. Alveolus
4. Oxygen
5. Carbon dioxide
6. Diffuse
7. Expired

IV. GASES ARE TRANSPORTED BY THE CIRCULATORY SYSTEM
1. Oxygen
2. Hemoglobin
3. Bicarbonate ions
4. Plasma

V. RESPIRATION IS REGULATED BY THE BRAIN
1. Respiratory centers

2. Breathing
3. Forcefully
4. Respiratory failure
5. Cellular respiration; Ventilation
6. Chemoreceptors
7. Blood
8. Oxygen
9. Hyperventilate
10. Cardiopulmonary resuscitation

VI. THE RESPIRATORY SYSTEM DEFENDS ITSELF AGAINST POLLUTED AIR

1. Respiratory
2. Hair; Mucous lining
3. Bronchial
4. Cilia
5. Macrophages
6. Lymph
7. Carbon
8. Disease
9. Lung

Figure 14-1: See Figure 14-1 in your textbook.

CHAPTER TEST

1. c
2. b
3. c
4. b
5. d
6. d
7. b
8. a
9. d
10. b
11. d
12. a
13. d

CHAPTER 15

STUDY QUESTIONS

INTRODUCTION

1. Nutrients
2. Energy
3. Nutrition
4. Digestive

I. THE DIGESTIVE SYSTEM PROCESSES FOOD

1. Ingestion
2. Digestion
3. Mechanical
4. Chemical
5. Absorption
6. Elimination
7. Liver

II. THE DIGESTIVE SYSTEM CONSISTS OF THE DIGESTIVE TRACT AND ACCESSORY ORGANS

1. Alimentary
2. Mouth; Anus
3. Gastrointestinal
4. Salivary; Liver; Pancreas
5. 3; 1; 4; 2; 6; 5

A. The Wall of the Digestive Tract Has Four Layers

1. Digestive
2. Mucosa; Epithelial
3. Digestion
4. Submucosa
5. Peristalsis
6. Connective
7. Parietal peritoneum
8. Peritoneal cavity
9. Peritonitis

B. Folds of the Peritoneum Support the Digestive Organs

1. Mesentery
2. Intestine
3. Peritoneum
4. Greater omentum
5. Lesser omentum
6. Mesocolon

C. The Mouth Ingests Food

1. Oral cavity
2. Mechanical
3. Tongue
4. Taste buds

1. The Teeth Break Down Food

1. Alveolar
2. Crown; Roots
3. Dentin
4. Enamel
5. Pulp cavity; Pulp
6. Root canals
7. Deciduous
8. Incisor
9. Canines

Figure 15-1: See Figure 15-4A in your textbook.

2. The Salivary Glands Produce Saliva

1. Parotid
2. Submandibular
3. Sublingual
4. Saliva; Salivary amylase
5. Bolus

D. The Pharynx Is Important in Swallowing

1. Swallowing
2. Pharynx

3. Oropharynx; Nasopharynx; Laryngopharynx
4. Soft palate
5. Hard palate
6. Uvula
7. Tongue
8. Esophagus
9. Epiglottis

E. The Esophagus Conducts Food to the Stomach
1. Pharynx
2. Stomach
3. Peristaltic
4. Sphincter
5. Esophagus
6. Heartburn

F. The Stomach Digests Food
1. Cardiac; Stomach
2. Rugae
3. Contractions
4. Peristalsis
5. Mucus
6. Glands
7. Pepsinogen
8. Chyme
9. Pyloric
10. Small intestine

G. Most Digestion Takes Place in the Small Intestine
1. Small intestine
2. Duodenum
3. Jejunum; Ileum
4. Villi
5. Absorption
6. Digestion
7. Intestinal glands
8. Goblet cells
9. Pancreas

H. The Pancreas Secretes Enzymes
1. Pancreas
2. Exocrine
3. Pancreatic juice; Enzymes
4. Duodenum
5. Acute pancreatitis

I. The Liver Secretes Bile
1. Liver
2. Liver cell
3. Lobe
4. Hepatic
5. Portal
6. Intestine
7. Bile

8. Gallbladder
9. Common bile duct

III. DIGESTION OCCURS AS FOOD MOVES THROUGH THE DIGESTIVE TRACT
1. Chyme
2. Gastrin
3. Reflexes

A. Glucose Is the Main Product of Carbohydrate Digestion
1. Glucose
2. Mouth
3. Salivary amylase; Maltose
4. Pancreatic amylase
5. Maltase
6. Sucrose; Lactose
7. Carbohydrate

B. Bile Emulsifies Fat
1. Duodenum
2. Bile
3. Lipase
4. Triglycerides; Fatty acids; Glycerol

C. Proteins Are Digested to Free Amino Acids
1. Amino acids
2. Peptide
3. Protein
4. Stomach; Pepsin
5. Polypeptides
6. Trypsin

IV. THE INTESTINAL VILLI ABSORB NUTRIENTS
1. Villi
2. Villus
3. Lacteal
4. Absorbed
5. Liver
6. Fatty acids

V. THE LARGE INTESTINE ELIMINATES WASTES
1. Chyme
2. Ileocecal
3. Peristaltic
4. Cecum
5. Vermiform appendix
6. Appendicitis
7. Colon
8. Ascending colon
9. Transverse colon
10. Sigmoid colon; Rectum
11. Anal canal
12. Feces
13. Defecate

VI. A BALANCED DIET IS NECESSARY TO MAINTAIN HEALTH

1. Energy sources
2. Water
3. Minerals
4. Vitamins
5. Carbohydrates
6. Lipids
7. Proteins
8. Essential amino acids
9. Oxidants
10. Antioxidants

VII. ENERGY METABOLISM IS BALANCED WHEN ENERGY INPUT EQUALS ENERGY OUTPUT

1. Metabolic rate
2. Heat
3. Basal metabolic rate
4. Total metabolic rate
5. Stored fat; Decreases
6. Malnutrition

7. Obesity

Figure 15-2: See Figure 15-1 in your textbook.

CHAPTER TEST

1. b
2. d
3. d
4. d
5. a
6. c
7. b
8. a
9. d
10. a
11. d
12. c
13. d
14. c
15. d
16. b
17. b

SOLUTION TO CROSSWORD PUZZLE FOR CHAPTERS 14 AND 15

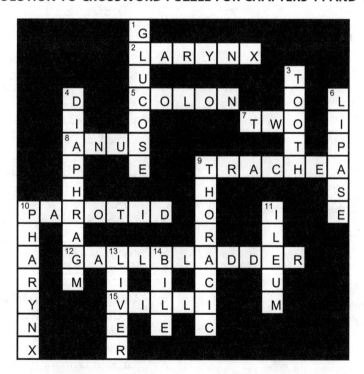

CHAPTER 16

STUDY QUESTIONS

INTRODUCTION

1. Urinary
2. Water
3. Homeostatic
4. Excesses

5. Excretion
6. Elimination

I. METABOLIC WASTE PRODUCTS INCLUDE WATER, CARBON DIOXIDE, AND NITROGENOUS WASTES

1. Nitrogenous wastes
2. Nitrogen
3. Ammonia; Urea
4. Uric acid

5. Kidneys
6. Sweat glands
7. Urine
8. Lungs
9. Liver; Hemoglobin

II. THE URINARY SYSTEM HAS MANY REGULATORY FUNCTIONS

1. Urine
2. Excretes
3. Blood; Body fluids
4. Renin
5. Erythropoietin

III. THE URINARY SYSTEM CONSISTS OF THE KIDNEYS, URINARY BLADDER, AND THEIR DUCTS

1. Kidneys
2. Urine
3. Bladder; Ureters
4. Urinary bladder
5. Urethra

A. The Kidneys Consist of a Cortex and Medulla

1. Retroperitoneal
2. Renal artery; Renal vein
3. Kidney
4. Hilus
5. Renal capsule
6. Cortex; Medulla
7. Renal papilla
8. Calyx
9. Major calyx
10. Renal pelvis
11. 3; 4; 5; 1; 2

B. The Nephrons Are the Functional Units of the Kidney

1. Nephrons
2. Urine
3. Corpuscle; Filtrate; Tubule
4. Blood; Collecting ducts
5. Glomerulus; Bowman's capsule
6. Afferent arteriole; Efferent arteriole
7. Peritubular
8. Juxtaglomerular
9. 3; 5; 1; 4; 2

C. Urine Is Transported by Ducts and Stored in the Bladder

1. Ureters
2. Peristaltic
3. Urinary bladder
4. Urethra
5. Prostate; Penis
6. Vagina
7. Bladder

D. Urination Empties the Bladder

1. Micturition
2. Urination reflex
3. External urethral sphincter
4. Nervous system
5. Urinate

IV. URINE IS PRODUCED BY FILTRATION, REABSORPTION, AND SECRETION

1. Glomerular; Tubular reabsorption; Tubular secretion

A. Glomerular Filtration Is Not Selective With Regard to Small Molecules and Ions

1. Glomerular filtration
2. Kidney; Glomerular filtrate
3. Blood plasma
4. Glucose; Amino acids
5. Blood cells; Proteins
6. Body

B. Tubular Reabsorption Is Highly Selective

1. Tubular reabsorption
2. Renal tubules; Ducts
3. Selective
4. Urine

C. Some Substances Are Secreted From the Blood Into the Filtrate

1. Tubular secretion; Renal tubules
2. Creatinine
3. Homeostatic
4. Penicillin

D. Urine Consists Mainly of Water

1. Renal pelvis
2. Urine
3. Water; Nitrogenous wastes; Salts
4. Sterile
5. Bacterial action
6. Ammonia

V. URINE VOLUME AND COMPOSITION ARE REGULATED BY HORMONES

1. Kidney
2. Dehydrate
3. Greater; Osmotic pressure
4. Hypothalamus
5. ADH
6. Diabetes insipidus
7. Aldosterone
8. Diuretics
9. Reabsorption

VI. THE VOLUME AND COMPOSITION OF BODY FLUID MUST BE REGULATED

1. Water

2. Blood plasma; Lymph; Interstitial fluid (any order)
3. Chemical reactions
4. Transport

A. The Body Has Two Main Fluid Compartments
1. Intracellular; Extracellular
2. Cells
3. Volume
4. Blood pressure; Osmotic
5. Lymphatic

B. Fluid Intake Must Equal Fluid Output
1. Fluid output
2. Ingested
3. Metabolism
4. Kidneys
5. Dehydration
6. Hypothalamus
7. Thirst center

C. Electrolyte Balance and Fluid Balance Are Interdependent
1. Electrolytes
2. Ions
3. Nonelectrolytes
4. Glucose; Urea
5. Cations
6. Anions
7. Electrolyte balance

D. Electrolytes Serve Vital Functions
1. Sodium
2. Nervous; Muscle
3. Coma
4. Water
5. Aldosterone
6. Potassium
7. Acid-base
8. Heart failure
9. Urine
10. Phosphate
11. Chloride
12. Osmotic pressure
13. Magnesium

VII. ACID-BASE BALANCE MUST BE MAINTAINED
1. Acid-base
2. pH
3. Neutral
4. Higher; Acidity
5. Lower; Alkalinity
6. Basic
7. Blood
8. Acidosis

9. Alkalosis
10. Chemical buffer
11. Bicarbonate; Phosphate; Protein
12. Hemoglobin
13. Respiratory acidosis
14. Respiratory alkalosis

Figure 16-1: See Figure 16-2 in your textbook.
Figure 16-2: See Figure 16-4 in your textbook.

CHAPTER TEST
1. b
2. d
3. b
4. a
5. b
6. c
7. b
8. b
9. c
10. b
11. a
12. d
13. c
14. d
15. b
16. d
17. a

CHAPTER 17

STUDY QUESTIONS

INTRODUCTION
1. Reproduction
2. Gametes
3. Lactation
4. Gonads

I. THE MALE PRODUCES SPERM
1. Sperm
2. Egg; Sex
3. Testes; Scrotum; Penis

A. The Testes Produce Sperm and Hormones
1. Testes
2. Seminiferous
3. Spermatogenesis
4. Chromosomes
5. Sperm
6. Scrotum
7. Inguinal
8. Inguinal hernia

B. The Conducting Tubes Transport Sperm
1. Epididymis
2. Vas deferens

3. Spermatic cord
4. Ejaculatory
5. Urethra
6. Sperm; Urine
7. 3; 5; 1; 2; 4

C. The Accessory Glands Produce Semen
1. Semen
2. Prostate
3. Bulbourethral
4. Ejaculation
5. Sperm cells
6. Sterile

D. The Penis Delivers Sperm Into the Female Reproductive Tract
1. Penis
2. Shaft; Glans
3. Prepuce
4. Circumcision
5. Corpus; Sinusoids
6. Erect
7. Ejaculation
8. Reflex

E. Hormones Regulate Male Reproduction
1. Androgens
2. Testosterone
3. Development
4. Primary
5. Secondary
6. Puberty
7. Hypothalamus; Gonadotropic
8. Follicle stimulating hormone (FSH)
9. Luteinizing hormone (LH)
10. Negative feedback

Figure 17-1: See Figure 17-1 in your textbook.
Figure 17-2: See Figure 17-2 in your textbook.

II. THE FEMALE PRODUCES OVA AND INCUBATES THE EMBRYO
1. Ova; Sperm
2. Menstrual cycle
3. Ovaries
4. Uterus
5. Vagina

A. The Ovaries Produce Ova and Hormones
1. Ovaries
2. Ova; Estrogen; Progesterone
3. Ovarian
4. Oogenesis
5. Follicle
6. Puberty
7. Female hormones
8. Graafian

9. Ovulation
10. Corpus luteum

B. The Uterine Tubes Transport Ova
1. Oviduct; Fallopian
2. Fimbriae
3. Pelvic
4. Uterus
5. Fertilization
6. Zygote
7. Ovum

C. The Uterus Incubates the Embryo
1. Uterus
2. Embryo
3. Menstruation
4. Corpus
5. Fundus
6. Cervix
7. Endometrium
8. Papanicolaou (Pap)

D. The Vagina Functions in Sexual Intercourse, Menstruation, and Birth
1. Vagina
2. Endometrium
3. Cervix
4. Fornices
5. Collapsed; Rugae
6. Enlarging

E. The External Genital Structures Are the Vulva
1. Vulva
2. Mons pubis
3. Puberty
4. Labia majora
5. Labia minora
6. Clitoris
7. Vestibule
8. Urethra; Vagina
9. Hymen
10. Bartholin's
11. Clinical perineum

F. The Breasts Contain the Mammary Glands
1. Lactation
2. Breasts
3. Ligaments of Cooper
4. Milk
5. Nipple
6. Colostrum
7. Prolactin
8. Oxytocin
9. Lymphatic
10. Mammography

G. Hormones Regulate Female Reproduction
1. Progesterone
2. Estrogens
3. Puberty
4. Menarche
5. Menstrual cycle
6. Ovulation
7. Menstruation
8. LH
9. Menopause
10. Estrogen replacement

Figure 17-3: See Figure 17-4 in your textbook.
Figure 17-4: See Figure 17-5 in your textbook.

III. FERTILIZATION IS THE FUSION OF SPERM AND OVUM
1. Uterus
2. Fertilization
3. Follicle
4. Ovum
5. Zygote
6. Ejaculation
7. Ovulation

IV. THE ZYGOTE GIVES RISE TO THE NEW INDIVIDUAL
1. Zygote
2. Embryo
3. Uterine tube; Cilia
4. Uterus

A. The Embryo Develops in the Wall of the Uterus
1. Uterus
2. Fetal
3. Amnion
4. Placenta
5. Blood
6. Progesterone
7. Human chorionic gonadotropin (hCG)
8. Umbilical cord

B. Prenatal Development Requires About 266 Days
1. Menstrual period
2. Brain; Spinal cord
3. Limb buds
4. Fetus
5. Fetal movements
6. Cerebrum
7. Lanugo
8. Premature

C. The Birth Process Includes Labor and Delivery
1. Parturition
2. Labor
3. First stage
4. Dilated; Effaced
5. Amnion; Amniotic
6. Second stage; Delivery
7. Placenta
8. Third stage
9. Afterbirth

D. Multiple Births May Be Fraternal or Identical
1. Fertility
2. Fraternal
3. Identical
4. Genes
5. Conjoined

V. THE HUMAN LIFE CYCLE EXTENDS FROM FERTILIZATION TO DEATH
1. Development
2. Neonatal
3. Infancy
4. Childhood
5. Adolescence
6. Young adulthood
7. Middle age
8. Old age

CHAPTER TEST
1. d
2. b
3. c
4. a
5. b
6. d
7. b
8. a
9. c
10. b
11. c
12. d
13. a
14. c
15. c
16. b
17. a
18. b
19. c
20. b

SOLUTION TO CROSSWORD PUZZLE FOR CHAPTERS 16 AND 17

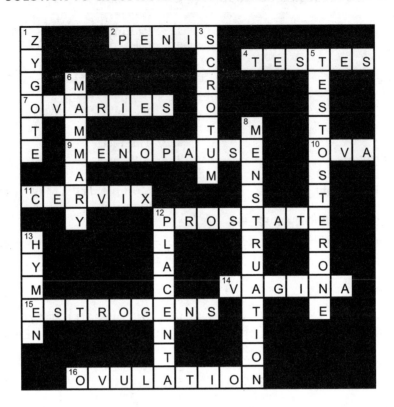